M000236038

Selecting the Proper Products for Your Skin

The acne aisle at the drug store is huge, and it can be confusing! So if you're taking the over-the-counter route to treating your acne, check out the following table to find out which type of acne-fighting product may work well for you. The *base* is simply the inactive ingredient that holds the medication.

Base	Best for This Skin	Description
Alcohol solutions	Oily	Evaporate quickly. The most drying of all these treatments and can be very irritating. Cover large areas easily.
Aqueous solutions	Normal to dry	Water based and alcohol-free. Less drying and irritating than alcohol solutions. Cover large areas easily.
Creams	Normal to oily	Generally more popular than ointments because they're less greasy. Often preferred by patients because they absorb into the skin quickly. Their water content makes them more drying than ointments.
Foams	Normal to oily	May be somewhat drying, but they're easy to spread, particularly on hairy areas such as chests and backs of males. Very expensive.
Gels	Normal to oily	Essentially oil-free and have a mildly drying effect. Some of the newer gel preparations contain emollients such as glycerin and dimethicone, which help diminish the drying effects.
Lotions	Any	May be somewhat moisturizing; however, those that contain propylene glycol may have drying effects. Easy to apply.
Ointment	Normal to dry	Greasy. More lubricating and tend to be less irritating than creams and gels.

For Dummies: Bestselling Book Series for Beginners

Acne For Dummies®

Getting Down to Business with Your Dermatologist

Whether you're seeing your primary healthcare provider or your dermatologist for the first time about your acne, spend a few minutes getting ready so that you can give your doctor all the information he needs to help you formulate the best treatment plan.

Know your *medical history*, which includes information on the following:

- Current medications
- Other medical problems
- Allergies
- Other skin conditions
- Vitamins and supplements

The following are my typical *first-visit questions* about acne. To ensure that you don't forget anything, **spend a few minutes thinking about these questions before the visit:**

- How long have you had acne?
- Does it run in your family?
- Is there anyone in the family with severe scarring acne?
- What do you do to your skin each day?
- Do you pick at lesions?
- What seems to make it worse? Diet, exercise, medications, stress?
- What has been helpful? Sunlight, vacations, medications, winning the lottery?

And if you're a female, you'll also get these old standbys:

- Does it get worse before your period or at midcycle?
- Does makeup make it worse?
- Are your periods normal?
- Are you taking birth control pills and do they seem to help or worsen your acne?
- Have you noticed any unusual or excessive hair growth?

On the *day of your visit*, keep the following in mind:

- Arrive 15 minutes early if you're a new patient to allow time for paperwork.
- Bring a parent or guardian if you're under 18.
- Bring your insurance card.
- Remove any makeup before your visit.

Copyright © 2006 Wiley Publishing, Inc.
All rights reserved.
Item 4698-3.
For more information about Wiley Publishing, call 1-800-762-2974.

For Dummies: Bestselling Book Series for Beginners

Acne

FOR
DUMMIES®

by Herbert P. Goodheart, MD

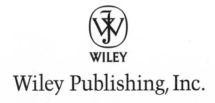

WILEY

Wiley Publishing, Inc.

WILEY

About the Author

Herbert P. Goodheart, MD, has been in the private practice of dermatology for over 25 years. He is a fellow of the American Academy of Dermatology and a member of the Greater New York Dermatological Society. For 20 years, Dr. Goodheart was an Assistant Clinical Professor of Medicine in the Division of Dermatology at the Albert Einstein College of Medicine, Bronx, New York, and is now an Assistant Clinical Professor in the Department of Dermatology at the Mount Sinai College of Medicine in New York City.

Dr. Goodheart is the author of *Goodheart's Photoguide of Common Skin Disorders, Diagnosis and Management,* a clinical guide to assist the primary care provider and dermatologist-in-training in the identification and treatment of common skin disorders. The book, which is in its second edition, was a unanimous choice for first prize in dermatology at the annual British Medical Association Book Awards for 2004.

He also is a contributing editor of *Women's Health in Primary Care,* a medical journal for physicians and other healthcare professionals. Dr. Goodheart's monthly column, "Dermatology Rounds," provides information on the wide spectrum of skin disorders affecting women.

He lives in New York City with his wife Karen and his son David.

Dedication

This book is dedicated to my parents, Nathan and Rose Goodheart, who instilled in me the importance of something they were deprived of — a good education. Their love, sacrifices, and encouragement have allowed me to pursue my career in medicine. I also dedicate it to my beloved sister and brother Myra Krenzel and Bernie Goodheart. My love and thanks also go to my in-laws, Dr. Norman Schneeberg and Helen Schneeberg, who have been supportive of me all along the way and who allowed me to marry their daughter, Karen.

Author's Acknowledgments

This project proved to be far from a solo effort. Mike Baker, the project editor, was at my side throughout the entire project. With his steadfast patience, attention to detail, and great intelligence, he was a true partner in bringing this complicated project to completion. Thank you Mike — I really enjoyed working with you! The great acquisitions editor, Kathy Cox, deserves credit for her wonderful guidance in always keeping the book on course. Special thanks goes to Heather Dismore who was an indispensable support in helping me overcome some difficult obstacles. Jen Bingham, my copy editor, made many suggestions that were right on target and helped to make *Acne For Dummies* both clear and concise. I also want to thank the talented group at Wiley, including my illustrator, Kathryn Borne, and the entire production staff. They all deserve huge praise!

A big thanks to Linda Roghaar, my literary agent, who brought me to *For Dummies* and helped make this book a reality. My deep gratitude goes to my friends Jane Friedman Century and Richard Lieberman for their inspiration and helpful suggestions. I also wish to thank my dermatologist friends and colleagues, Drs. Hendrik Uyttendaele, Ross Levy, Diane Berson, Ron Shelton, and Peter Burk, for their assistance in working through difficult problems.

I deeply appreciate the efforts of my technical editor, Joe Eastern, MD, whose watchful eye assured the scientific and clinical integrity of the text. Also I would like to thank Sandra Mamis, RPA-C, physician assistant *par excellence,* who helped to review some of my difficult chapters, Ilene Buchalter, who knows how to run a dermatology office and helped me to describe it, and Lance Brown, MD, who provided me with material about acne scars.

Many thanks go to my colleagues at Derm-Chat/Derm-Rx, who keep me up to date on the latest diagnostic and therapeutic issues in dermatology. Art Huntley, MD, at UC Davis, who founded and maintains this valuable online resource, deserves special credit. I also am indebted to my patients who taught me more than anyone about acne.

Special love and appreciation go to *ma belle soeur,* Susan Bronstein, whose foresight was the driving force behind my pursuing *Acne For Dummies.* When she heard about *For Dummies,* she immediately thought of me. Also, a big hug and kiss goes to my 14-year-old son, David, who proofread the chapters on teenage acne and gave me tremendous computer assistance. Most of all, I wish to thank my wife Karen for her support, encouragement, and great editing. Her skills and patience helped me throughout the long journey that led to this publication.

Publisher's Acknowledgments

We're proud of this book; please send us your comments through our Dummies online registration form located at www.dummies.com/register/.

Some of the people who helped bring this book to market include the following:

Acquisitions, Editorial, and Media Development

Project Editor: Mike Baker

Acquisitions Editor: Kathleen M. Cox

Copy Editor: Jennifer Bingham

Technical Reviewer: Joseph Eastern, MD

Editorial Manager: Christine Meloy Beck

Editorial Assistants: David Lutton, Hanna Scott

Cartoons: Rich Tennant (www.the5thwave.com)

Composition Services

Project Coordinator: Erin Smith

Layout and Graphics: Carl Byers, Joyce Haughey, Stephanie D. Jumper, Lynsey Osborn

Special Art: Illustrations, Kathryn Born; Photos, Herbert P. Goodheart and *Goodheart's Photoguide of Common Skin Disorders,* Sonya Seigafus, ed., Lippincott Williams & Wilkins, 2003.

Proofreaders: Leeann Harney, Carl Pierce, Charles Spencer, TECHBOOKS Production Services

Indexer: TECHBOOKS Production Services

Publishing and Editorial for Consumer Dummies

    Diane Graves Steele, Vice President and Publisher, Consumer Dummies

    Joyce Pepple, Acquisitions Director, Consumer Dummies

    Kristin A. Cocks, Product Development Director, Consumer Dummies

    Michael Spring, Vice President and Publisher, Travel

    Kelly Regan, Editorial Director, Travel

Publishing for Technology Dummies

    Andy Cummings, Vice President and Publisher, Dummies Technology/General User

Composition Services

    Gerry Fahey, Vice President of Production Services

    Debbie Stailey, Director of Composition Services

Contents at a Glance

Table of Contents

Chapter 17: Coping with the Psychological Scars . . . 203

Chapter 18: Reining in Rosacea and Other Acne Look-Alikes 211

Chapter 19: Fighting the Feisty Follicle. 229

Introduction

- -

*A*cne — it's not exactly a subject that you like to talk about every day. At social events, you do your best to conceal it under makeup (although if you're a man, makeup is usually not a realistic option). For kids, acne is more than just a stage of adolescence — it's the pits! In fact, acne can be a problem for people of any age. Even newborns and seniors can develop acne!

Americans currently spend more than $4 billion a year on skin treatments, nearly $100 million of which goes toward nonprescription acne medications alone. We lavish millions on expensive special soaps and cleansers, prescription therapies, and visits to physicians. Besides money, we also spend an enormous amount of time at beauty counters, salons, spas, and tanning parlors.

Much of this extravagance is encouraged by the messages we get from the media that market unrealistic promises. Ad campaigns promote skin care products using models and movie stars that have perfect, radiant skin. They perpetuate the idea that clear, youthful appearing skin is the only way to go; imperfections are to be looked down on as something to be ashamed of. Many myths and misconceptions about skin care in general, and acne specifically, continue to be widely believed.

During my 25 years of practicing dermatology, I've observed my patients trying to cope with the embarrassment of acne and related skin disorders. That's what motivated me to write a realistic, practical guide for the understanding and treatment of acne and related conditions. My goal is to dispel many of the myths and misconceptions and to help the reader find out more about his or her condition and manage it more successfully.

Keep in mind that attractiveness to others is much more than physical beauty. It also includes such factors as intelligence and personality. Remember — beauty and acne are only skin deep!

About This Book

Acne For Dummies is intended as a reference for people who have teenage acne, adult acne, and other acnelike conditions such as rosacea and razor bumps.

When I reviewed the existing books on acne that are intended for the general public, I discovered that most of them offer limited, and at times misleading, information. Many adopt a self-serving manner selling products or trying to prove that their point of view is the acne "cure."

Although some of these books describe well-accepted therapies, others promise results that can't be realistically delivered, and are based solely upon the authors' opinions without any credible research to back up their claims. Furthermore, these publications often fail to address African-Americans and other minority groups; they're targeted to a white, mostly adult-female, audience.

This book is intended to have a wide appeal to readers of all ages: teens and their parents, women and men of all ages, persons of color and of various ethnic backgrounds. I also want it to serve as a source of information for pediatricians, primary care providers, physician assistants, nurse practitioners, school nurses, school librarians, healthcare providers in the military, and anyone else who cares for people with acne and related disorders.

Conventions Used in This Book

To help you find your way in this book, I use the following conventions:

- ✓ Web page addresses appear in `monofont`.
- ✓ *Italics* are used both for emphasis and to point out new words or terms that are defined.
- ✓ **Bold** highlights the keywords in bulleted lists or action parts of numbered steps.
- ✓ Sidebars, which look like text enclosed in a shaded gray box, consist of information that's interesting to know but not necessarily critical to your understanding of the chapter or section's topic.

Foolish Assumptions

Every author has to make some assumptions about his audience, and I'm not any different. So, I assume that:

- ✓ You or someone you know has acne or an acnelike condition. (How's that for a wild guess?)
- ✓ You want to know more about how to treat acne on your own.

✔ You want a concise and easy-to-understand guide to over-the-counter and prescription acne medications and treatment options. You want to know what works and what doesn't.

✔ You want to find simple, clear explanations about caring for your skin without all the hype.

✔ You're looking for information on acnelike conditions, such as rosacea and razor bumps.

✔ You're a healthcare provider who's looking for an easy-to-use reference for yourself and your patients.

Well, if one or more of these descriptions sounds about right, you've come to the right place.

How This Book Is Organized

Acne For Dummies is organized into seven major parts — the following sections give a quick rundown on what you'll find in each of them. You don't have to read this book cover to cover (although I wouldn't mind if you did). You can just jump in anywhere you like because each section is self-contained.

Part I: Facing Up to Acne

In Part I of this book, I give you the essentials of acne: its definition, its causes, its appearance, how it arises in your skin, and whom it affects. I also provide you with some general information about the scene of the crime — your skin — and how to determine whether you should treat it on your own or call on a doctor.

Part II: Figuring Out Your Acne and How to Tackle It on Your Own

Here you find that not all acne is alike; in fact, you discover all skin isn't alike. Acne has many faces and different features in both sexes and in the various age groups. In Chapter 4, I talk about teenage acne; Chapter 5 explores acne in adults; and in Chapter 6, I discuss the factors that may or may not make your acne worse. Finally, in Chapter 7, I provide you with a complete guide to over-the-counter acne-fighting preparations.

Part III: Turning to the Pros to Treat Your Type of Acne

Part III is loaded with an abundant supply of information tailored to focus on the right professional treatment for all types of acne. I start off by helping you find a dermatologist or other medical professional to help you get your treatment underway. Then I discuss the many choices you have among medications, lights, lasers, and surgery, as well as alternative methods to treat acne. Discussions of acne in teens, adults, folks with dark complexions, the elderly, the very young, and the expectant mother — they're all here.

Part IV: Dealing with Scars and Associated Conditions

In this part, I get physical and emotional. I give you tips on how to treat acne scars based on the kinds of scars you have *and* the kind of skin you have. Because acne can be so emotionally devastating, I also delve into the emotional hurdles that you or your friends and family have to contend with and how to help avoid, manage, and prevent them. I help you figure out when to seek professional help and what treatments might be right for you.

I then complete the picture with skin conditions that look like acne — the acne impersonators such as rosacea and pseudofolliculitis (shaving bumps). I also tell you what symptoms may suggest an associated hormonal disorder.

Part VI: The Part of Tens

The parts of tens are a mainstay feature of *For Dummies* books. In this grouping of top ten lists, I go over ten terrific Web sites where you can find additional reliable information about acne and rosacea. You can also find my top ten tips for keeping your skin looking its best. And finally, I include my ten recommendations for things to never, ever do to, for, or with your skin.

Part VII: Appendixes

The appendixes in this book are intended to be helpful for you as you come across information that's not familiar. I included a glossary so that you can look up jargony words that are part of the acne world. Here you'll find terms your dermatologist uses, unfamiliar terms that are on the carton of your over-the-counter acne medicines, and even some that are on the TV commercials we all get to see while we're watching *The OC, Desperate Housewives,* or whatever programs geared toward teens or adult women might be on. I define each word when I use it the first time, but you may find it easier to check the glossary if you're skipping through the book.

I also have an appendix that lists all the medications I cover throughout this book and includes the various brand names that acne and rosacea drugs can go under in different countries.

Icons Used in This Book

The cute little round pictures that you see in the margins are like road signs that tell you about the things you should pay attention to while you're reading or browsing this book. They also tell you about the material you can avoid reading because it goes into too much technical detail.

This icon points out important information. It's the real "take home" stuff. Even, if you miss what's above or below, keep these tidbits in mind.

These chunks of information are helpful hints to really help you take better care of your skin and, sometimes, your pocketbook. This information is useful and important.

This icon indicates that there's lots of jargon and extra material. It's not critical and you can skip it if you're not very interested. On the other hand, if you're a budding dermatologist or just like technical, jargony bits, definitely don't skip 'em. It's your call.

This icon alerts you to things that you should avoid or be very cautious about — stuff that can be harmful to your health or your bank account. Definitely pay attention to this advice!

This icon tells you when you should give your healthcare professional a call.

Where to Go from Here

Where you start in this book completely depends on you. If you need to figure out what kind of acne you have, definitely go to Part II. If you're interested in how these pesky little zits form, Chapter 3 is a must-read. If you only want to look at treatment options, skip to Part III. If your acne has cleared up, but you want to manage and improve the lingering scars, check out Chapter 17. As with any *For Dummies* book, you can skip around and read what's important to you at any given time.

Part I
Facing Up to Acne

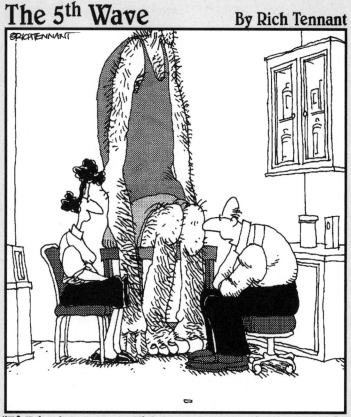

"If I had to guess, I'd say your son's acne is the result of a sudden surge of hormones."

In this part . . .

This is the place to start for the full story on acne. I give you an overview of the condition — its causes and appearance — and provide a few pointers on determining if you can treat it yourself with over-the-counter products or if it's time to call in a dermatologist. Then, I introduce you to the parts and functions of your skin, along with tips on caring for this vital organ. Finally, I walk you through the lifecycle of a pimple, explaining how acne forms.

Chapter 1

Dealing with Acne

In This Chapter

▶ Putting your best face forward

▶ Outlining treatment options

▶ Seeking the cure

▶ Looking at the look-alikes

*B*enjamin Franklin said, "In this world nothing can be said to be certain, except death and taxes," to which I would add a third certainty — acne. Acne is one of those equally dreaded, nearly universal experiences through which most of us pass during our teen years and, more recently, is increasingly coming back to revisit many of us as adults. In this chapter, you find out that you're not alone in your desire to have clear skin. Along the way, you discover that acne is a treatable condition and many of the treatment options are made to order for your type of acne.

Acne Explained

Acne is the most common skin disorder in the world. *Blemishes, bumps, papules, pustules, spots, whiteheads, zits, goobers, the plague,* or whatever you call it, almost everyone is liable to get it. In the United States and Canada, acne affects 45 to 55 million individuals at some point in their lives, the vast majority of whom are teenagers. In fact, nearly 80 percent of all young people will face at least an occasional breakout of acne. Acne imposes itself on young men and young women about equally, but young men are likelier to have more severe forms of acne.

The events that take place in the sebaceous glands and hair follicles trigger acne. The exact cause is unknown; however, regardless of a person's age, acne is a condition of clogged hair follicles and the reaction of *sebaceous glands,* glands that are attached to hair follicles and produce an oily substance called *sebum.* Mix in some dead skin cells that become "sticky" and block the pores, add a bit of bacteria, and you have the makings of a breakout. For the full story on your skin, check out Chapter 2. And for a more detailed description about how pimples form, see Chapter 3.

Doctors believe that these events, and acne itself, result from several related factors, including your hormones (which are responsible for increasing oil production) and heredity (the tendency to develop acne is often inherited from parents and other relatives).

Less commonly, acne can occur as a reaction to certain drugs and chemicals, and other physical factors may exacerbate the problem. I cover all of these issues, including the myths and misinformation concerning the causes of acne, in Chapter 6 (and I review several hormonal disorders that can result in acne in Chapter 20), but I'll put one myth to bed right now that will come as good news.

Pizza, French fries, and other greasy foods don't cause acne or make it worse. You're welcome. (I'm a doctor, so I'm compelled to remind you that though these foods won't affect your acne, they aren't the building blocks of a healthy diet.) But before you snidely bring this mistaken notion to your mom's attention, another one of her common statements is right on the money: "Quit playing with your face." Picking does make zits worse!

Waking up to whiteheads, blackheads, and zits

In most cases, acne starts between the ages of 10 and 13 and usually lasts for 5 to 10 years. The appearance of teenage acne (*acne vulgaris* is the technical term that I throw around here and there in the book) is largely the result of your body's increased production of hormones. The good news is that those embarrassing blemishes usually go away and are often gone for good by the time you reach your early 20s.

However, the not-so-good news is that for some unlucky folks, acne vulgaris can persist into their late 20s or 30s or even beyond. But back to the good news: There are many steps you can take to zap the zits and improve the appearance of your skin, as I explain in the "Creating Your Acne-Treating Program" section, later in this chapter. And turn to Chapter 4 for the complete rundown on the causes, appearance, and other considerations of teenage acne.

Taking it on the chin later in life

Although acne is typically thought of as a condition of youth, an ever-growing number of women (less often men) get acne for the first time as adults. Acne is no longer just a teenage affliction. There's definitely been a rise in the number of adult women in their 20s and 30s with acne — even those who never had a pimple before!

Teenage and adult-onset acne have somewhat different characteristics. For one thing, the appearance is different: Adults have fewer blackheads and whiteheads; for another, adult acne tends to be more often located on the lower part of a woman's face. Also, the appearance of female adult-onset acne is often closely linked to a woman's menstrual cycle as well as increased sensitivity to hormones such as those brought about by pregnancy, starting or stopping birth control pills, and other hormonal abnormalities.

If you're really unlucky, you have adult-onset acne and have also brought along some acne vulgaris from your teenage years. I provide the full story on acne in adult women in Chapter 5.

Lights, camera, acne!

Whether you're a teenager who is noticing acne for the first time or an adult who anticipated permanently waving goodbye to it forever, you're in good company. The careers of Cameron Diaz, P. Diddy, Jessica Simpson, Alicia Keyes, Mike Myers, and Vanessa Williams have thrived despite their continuing complexion problems with acne.

And think about some of those rugged faces from the silver screen. From the looks of it, Tommy Lee Jones, Laurence Fishburne, Bill Murray, Edward James Olmos, James Woods, and the great British actor and movie star Richard Burton (who married Elizabeth Taylor, considered to be one of the most beautiful women in the world) more than likely had pretty wicked acne when they were teenagers.

Of course, heavy makeup, favorable lighting, medications, and experienced dermatologists have also probably helped them. I won't be able to supply your own personal makeup artist or a lighting technician to accompany you to school or work, but I do provide tons of recommendations on how to use acne-fighting medications and find a good dermatologist in this book.

You may not aspire to be a movie star. But the names I mention here are just a small number of the people who have achieved success in an area where looks count the most. Countless other people exist in all walks of life who went beyond their acne to become successes in their fields. And so can you.

Creating Your Acne-Treating Program

If you have acne in the 21st century, you're fortunate. Why? Because there are so many great ways to treat it and there are many more to come. But there are no quick cures for acne; in fact, there aren't really any cures. The goal of treatment is to manage your acne, help control it, prevent it from scarring, and help you look your best. The truth is that acne tends to heal itself over time, but the right therapy can make your skin look better.

Ye olde pimple remedies

For those of you who are squeamish or are dog lovers, skip to the next paragraph. Seventeenth-century Britons were as concerned about pimples as we are today. According to an old manuscript of home remedies that was recently discovered, people with acne were advised to cut the heads off two puppies, hang them up by their heels to bleed, collect the blood, mix the blood with white wine, and apply the concoction to the face. Yeech! Don't try it; it won't work!

At the beginning of the 20th century, most of the acne treatments involved the correction of intestinal disorders such as indigestion and constipation. Recommended anti-acne regimens included low-fat and low-sugar diets. Sound familiar? Excessive sweating was discouraged, and — get this — some doctors recommended that erotic preoccupation be avoided (without doubt, a difficult prescription to follow).

Active surgical treatment at that time included opening up and draining acne *lesions* (they're the zits), vigorous scrubbing, steaming, and washing with soap and hot water. All of this was followed by the application of foul-smelling chemicals including sulfur. For difficult-to-manage acne in middle-aged women, arsenic — both applied to the skin and injected into it — was sometimes used!

In the middle of the 20th century, when I was a teenager, I distinctly remember some of my fellow high school classmates coming to school with red, scaly faces the day after they visited their dermatologists. I've since learned that they were subjected to restrictive diets, carbon dioxide slush, superficial X-ray treatments, and ultraviolet light exposures, only to be followed by self-applied rigorous cleansings, scrubs, and chemical peeling agents. Ugh, no wonder their faces looked like red apples! It seems barbaric today, but that's all they had to treat acne at that time. Believe me, people who have acne today are much better off than when I was a teenager.

Meeting the players

Until the last couple of decades, there was very little anyone could do to treat acne. But we've now come a long way from the "dark ages" of arsenic and puppy blood (see the sidebar "Ye olde pimple remedies"). Now we have excellent methods to treat acne and the future looks even brighter. There are

- ✔ Over-the-counter *topical* (applied to the skin) products that contain such tried-and-true medicines as benzoyl peroxide (see Chapter 7 for a complete list of products, their pros and cons, and how to use them effectively)

- ✔ Topical antibiotics and retinoids (I discuss these in Chapter 9)

- ✔ Oral antibiotics (take a look at Chapter 10)

- ✔ Hormones and anti-androgens for females (see Chapter 11)

- ✔ Oral retinoids, like Accutane (see Chapter 13)

- ✔ Chemical peels, special lasers, and lights (see Chapter 14)

Some people also claim that various alternative and complementary approaches have helped improve their acne (in Chapter 15, I outline the possibilities and give you my input and advice on such matters).

Deciding whether to treat yourself

If you're just starting to get breakouts or you have really mild acne with a few blemishes here and there, the over-the-counter (OTC), do-it-yourself route that I describe in Chapter 7 may be just the ticket for you. Look in the mirror. If you see a few blackheads and whiteheads or a few pimples, you can probably find ways to treat them on your own.

You can find many acne products waiting for you at your local drugstores and cosmetic counters. You can do many things to improve the appearance of your skin without a prescription if you're a teenager just starting to get acne. Shelves are also stocked with products specifically geared toward adult women.

You can also follow some of my skin-care tips and further ideas to help you that I bring up throughout the book, like the face-washing advice I provide in Chapter 2, the tips for healthy skin in Chapter 22, or the list of things you should never do to your skin in Chapter 23.

Although going to a doctor generally costs more than buying a cream at your local drugstore, you'll likely save money in the long run and get better results than you'll get by running through the gamut of OTC acne products.

Relying on the experts

For some folks, acne can be more serious. In fact, by their mid-teens, more than 40 percent of adolescents have acne severe enough to require some treatment by a physician or a dermatologist who is an authority when it comes to acne. And adult women who are having problems getting their acne to respond to treatment often need to make an appointment with a doctor.

But no matter who you are, you should definitely have your acne evaluated by a knowledgeable healthcare provider if:

- ✔ Your acne didn't respond to home remedies, diets, herbal medications, facials, special soaps, or nonprescription OTC treatments.

- ✔ Your skin can't tolerate the OTC preparations.

- ✔ Your acne is widespread and it involves your chest and back.

- ✔ Your acne is beginning to scar or has already scarred.

- ✔ Your acne has become more severe.

- ✔ You are a female who develops facial hair or has irregular periods (I address this issue in Chapter 20).

- ✔ You're not a "do-it-yourselfer" and you want the pros to handle your acne.

- ✔ You have dark skin, and patches that are darker than your normal skin appear after your acne lesions clear. (For treatment considerations particular to folks with darker skin, turn to Chapter 12.)

In addition, you may need help dealing with acne scars, both the physical and emotional:

- ✔ **Preventing and repairing scars:** Even very mild or occasional breakouts have the potential to leave permanent scars. There are now exciting innovations in dermatologic surgery using lights, lasers, and chemical peels to help improve the appearance of the skin before and after acne has left its marks. (Check out Chapters 14 and 16 for more information.)

> ✔ **Healing the inner scars:** The emotional effects of acne haven't always been fully appreciated, but many studies have demonstrated its damaging psychological impact. Nowadays there is a much greater interest in preventing and healing the inner scars of acne. In Chapter 17, I talk about the psychological and social scars of acne.

Avoiding quickie, quacky cures

Because your acne appears on your face and everyone can see it, you may feel desperate to make it go away. But because it's not life threatening, you may feel reluctant or embarrassed to go to your healthcare provider about it. Certain people prey on that knowledge. They want to sell you expensive over-the-counter acne "cures" that don't do you any good, or get you to order them after watching testimonial-filled infomercials.

The people giving those acne "testimonials" on TV are almost always professional actors reading a script. And even those stories that are "real" generally mean nothing. You can always find one or two success stories while ignoring 99.9 percent of failures.

Even if it's on TV, on the radio, the Internet, or in magazines, that doesn't mean it's necessarily true. The world of acne fighting is filled with snake oils and false promises.

There are promises that guarantee "five day cures" for your acne, and there are the real slow pokes that state, "try this all time-tested home treatment for acne and have clearer blemish-free skin within 30 days of use." You can find many similar "cures" if you search the Internet, so check out Chapter 21 where I give you some roadmaps to some realistic acne advice you can find on the Web.

Also, check out www.quackwatch.com, a nonprofit organization whose purpose is to combat health-related frauds, myths, fads, and fallacies pertaining to health-related issues. Its primary focus is on quackery-related information.

Recognizing Impostors and Related Conditions

There are several skin conditions that appear to be acne, but that aren't acne at all. *Rosacea* and *keratosis pilaris* closely resemble acne, as does another acne look-alike, *pseudofolliculitis barbae* — also known as razor bumps. These conditions, among others, are pretenders that sometimes even fool doctors into thinking they're actually acne. There are many ways to control these acne impostors; in Chapters 18 and 19 I show you how to do it.

Chapter 2

Getting Comfortable with the Skin You're In

In This Chapter

▶ Peeling back the layers

▶ Finding ways to keep your skin in shape

Do you know what the biggest organ in your body is? It's not your brain, and it's not your large intestine. Give up? The subject of this book may have given the answer away, so I'll suspend any further guesswork and tell you: It's your skin. That's right; your skin is an organ (just like your heart, lungs, and liver). And if you spread out the skin of the average adult it would measure 20 square feet, about the size of a twin-sized bed sheet!

In this chapter, I cover the ins and outs of your skin so that you can see just where your acne originates. I acquaint you with the many functions that your "largest organ" performs and tell you a little about how to take care of it.

Exploring Your Largest Organ

You may not really think of the skin as an organ, like the heart and lungs. To many people, skin seems more like a simple cover to prevent their insides from falling out. An *organ* is a somewhat independent part of the human body that performs a specific function. Once you know that, you can see that the skin *is* an organ, because it performs the following specific functions (in addition to others):

✔ Protects your body from infection

✔ Serves as a waterproof barrier between you and the outside world

✔ Shields you from the sun's harmful rays

✔ Provides cushioning like a shock absorber that defends you from injury

✔ Insulates your body and keeps your temperature right around a cozy 98.6 degrees Fahrenheit (37 degrees Celsius)

✔ Acts as an energy reserve

✔ Alerts you to potential harm through your sensations of touch and pain

✔ Repairs itself (that's why cuts heal)

✔ Produces vitamin D

Because your skin has so many functions, you may not be surprised to discover that it also has a rather complicated structure with many working parts. It contains hairs that have their own oil glands and tiny muscles — I'll bet that you didn't know that hairs have muscles! Your skin has sensory nerves — hot, cold, touch, and pressure receptors. It also is home to blood vessels, lymph vessels, and sweat glands. Plus, your skin has microscopic pigment-producing cells, cells that work on your immunity, as well as cells that protect and replace themselves. With all that going on, you may be surprised that your skin doesn't have its own zip code.

Human skin is made up of three layers. First come the top two layers — the *epidermis* (the outside layer of skin that you can touch and see) and the *dermis* (which is located directly beneath the epidermis). Then comes the third, bottom fatty layer that the epidermis and dermis rest upon, which is called the *subcutaneous layer.*

The prefix *epi* means "upon" and *derm* means "skin," so, together, they form *epidermis* (upon the skin). And obviously, *dermis* means "skin." The prefix *sub* means "under" and *cutaneous* is another reference to "skin," so the word *subcutaneous* means "under the skin." (I guess they should have named it the "subdermis" if they wanted to be totally consistent.)

In the sections that follow, I take you on a guided tour of each of these layers. And like any good tour guide, I provide you with a map in Figure 2-1.

Getting above it all: Hey, your epidermis is showing!

Your epidermis is really strong. The majority of the cells that make up the epidermis are called keratinocytes. *Keratinocytes* are filled with an exceptionally tough, fibrous, protein known as *keratin.*

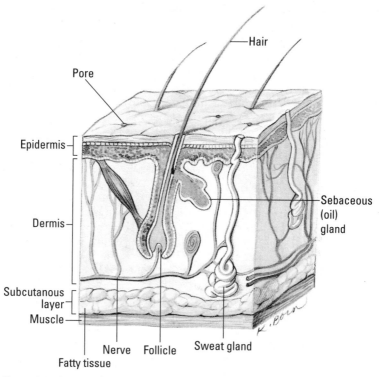

Figure 2-1: A cross section of your skin.

The Latin term for cells is "cytes." Therefore, *keratino-cytes,* by definition, are cells (cytes) comprised of keratin.

Just as your skin has more then one layer (epidermis, dermis, and subcutaneous layer), the epidermis itself has three layers. Within these layers, there's constant cellular motion going on.

✔ **Outer layer:** The outermost layer of the epidermis is known as the *stratum corneum,* also known as the *horny layer.* This layer provides your body with a durable overcoat that protects deeper cells from damage, infection, and from drying out.

This layer of your skin is actually made up of dead skin cells. (Your hair and nails are made of dead cells too!) So when you look at your skin, you're really seeing skin that is dead. But these deceased skin cells only stick around for a little while. Soon, they flake off — like when you wash, scratch yourself, go shopping, sit in class, fall asleep, and even read this book. Basically, all the time. In fact, every minute of the day we lose about 30,000 to 40,000 dead skin cells off the surface of our body.

✔ **Middle layer:** This layer is known as the *stratum spinosum.* The cells in this layer looked kind of spiny to the scientists who first described them.

✔ **Inner layer:** Known as the *basal layer,* the inner layer is like a production facility for the new skin cells (keratinocytes) that eventually make their way up through the stratum spinosum to the outer stratum corneum to replace the dead older cells you lose from the surface.

The keratinocytes in the basal layer stand up like little soldiers at attention on what's called the *basement membrane,* a barrier that separates the epidermis from the dermis; it's the anchor that joins the epidermis and dermis together. The keratinocytes are kept alive by the underlying dermis — which serves as their blood supply because the epidermis has no blood supply of its own. But their upward journey carries them farther away from their supply lines, and as they approach the top, they begin to die. By the time they've reached the outer layer of the epidermis, they've lost virtually all of their cellular contents except for tough keratin fibers and other solid proteins. Even as they dry up and die, they become much more resilient and durable and become the flattened cells that form the stratum corneum. This one-way trip takes about two weeks to a month to accomplish. Figure 2-2 demonstrates the process.

When an injury or an acne pimple penetrates the basement membrane, a scar may result. (I describe acne scarring in Chapter 16.)

Scratching the surface: Now your dermis is showing!

Your *dermis,* the layer of skin that lies just under your epidermis, has an intimate relationship with your epidermis. It comes equipped with sensory nerves, sweat glands, blood vessels, and hair follicles. It nourishes the epidermis by providing gases such as oxygen and carbon dioxide, which reach the epidermis by diffusing through the basement membrane. The epidermis can't survive without the dermis, because it has no nerves or blood supply of its own.

Throughout the dermis are collagen and elastin fibers. *Collagen* is a resilient protein that provides rigidity and strength to the dermis. *Elastin* is made of a protein structure that is able to coil and recoil like a spring. This protein is what gives the skin its elasticity.

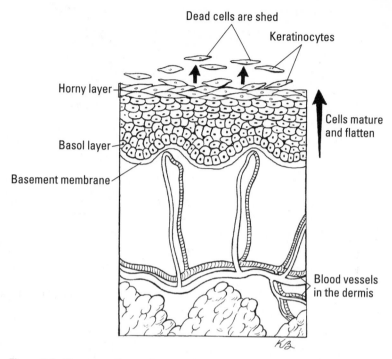

Figure 2-2: The maturation and upward migration of epidermal cells.

Also located in the dermis is the hair follicle (refer to Figure 2-1). A *hair follicle* is a hair-containing canal; a tube-shaped sheath that surrounds the part of the hair that is under the skin. It's located in the epidermis and the dermis. Blocked hair follicles are often at the root of the acne problem. In fact, it seems like the hair follicle is the central focus of this entire book! (To read a detailed description of how a follicle becomes blocked and a pimple forms, skip ahead to Chapter 3.)

Styes, boils, shaving bumps — I could go on and on — all have their origins in the hair follicle. In Chapter 19, I go into a few of these conditions that folks often mistake for acne.

Digging deeper: Your subcutaneous layer

Fat cells known as *lipocytes* reside in the subcutaneous layer. Our visit to the subcutaneous layer will be brief because as far as acne is concerned, there's not much action going on here.

The skinny on skin

Here are some skin facts you can use to impress your friends and family:

- ✔ Skin is your heaviest organ. It accounts for about 15 percent of your body weight. That means that the skin of a 400-pound sumo wrestler can weigh in at as much as 60 pounds! The skin of an average adult woman weighs about 20 pounds.

- ✔ The thickness of the average epidermis varies from 0.5 millimeters on your eyelids to 4.0 millimeters or more on the palms of your hands and the soles of your feet.

- ✔ You produce a totally new epidermis about every 30 days!

- ✔ Most of the dust in your classroom or bedroom is made of tiny fragments of human skin. In just one minute, 30,000 to 40,000 skin cells fall unseen from the surface of your body. That means you lose around 15 million or so skin cells in one year. (Imagine how dusty it must be in that sumo wrestler's bedroom!)

- ✔ Your dermis is several times thicker than the epidermis and is particularly thick on the upper back. Our thick upper back may have protected us from saber-toothed tigers when we walked on all fours. On second thought, I doubt it.

- ✔ "Goosebumps" come from tiny muscles called *erector pili*. These muscles attach to each of our hairs and make them stand at attention when we're cold or afraid. We can see this phenomenon on a frightened cat whose fur stands on end. It's meant to make kitty look bigger and scarier to other animals. And when we had more body hair during the Stone Age, it probably did the same for us.

- ✔ You have about 3 to 5 million hairs on your body.

- ✔ Your nails grow faster in warmer weather. They grow at a rate of 0.5 to 1.2 millimeters per day, with fingernails growing faster than toenails.

But if you're interested, your subcutaneous layer is what your outer layers of skin rest upon. Your fatty layer is your body's insulator, cushion, and natural shock absorber (and it also helps to keep the diet industry in business!). The subcutaneous layer contains arteries, veins, lymph vessels, and nerves that are larger than those found in your dermis. If you go any deeper, you'll come upon muscles and possibly some of your inner organs. That's out of bounds! So I'll end the anatomical tour right here in Fat City.

Basic Operating Instructions: Taking Care of Your Skin

Different people and different skin types need to do different things for their skin. We have an old expression in dermatology that still rings true: "If it's dry, wet it; if it's wet, dry it." In recent decades, another truism has been added: "If it's fair, shield it; if it's dark, you're probably very fortunate." That's because your melanin protects you from skin cancers, wrinkling, and keeps you looking young.

If your skin is fair, if you burn easily, or if you have a personal or family history of skin cancer, you should protect yourself from the sun by wearing hats and caps, using sunscreens, and avoiding going to tanning parlors. If your skin is dark, you may have other reasons to protect it from the sun (see Chapter 12 where I talk about the dark spots that occur in dark skin). People with dark complexioned or Asian skin may have other reasons to be very sensitive and prone to irritation and possibly less tolerant of many of the topical medications that are used to treat acne.

The ultimate operating instruction: Whether you have dry, regular, or oily skin, a big acne breakout or smooth sailing on the pimple front, there's something that'll keep your face looking its best and most attractive to the rest of the world and is guaranteed to help you make friends and influence people. I suggest that you simply exercise your muscles of facial expression — and smile!

Washing your face

Rocket science? Maybe not. But as a dermatologist, I have a few reasons for walking you through a little face-washing tutorial. First, I often begin my instructions for applying medications in later chapters with phrases like "Wash your skin . . ." or "To a clean, dry face, apply . . ." so, it seemed to make sense that I fill you in on the details. The second reason for this bit of Face Washing 101 is even simpler — many people screw it up. But don't worry: I'm here to help. And, if you're like many folks, my face-washing routine can simplify your mornings and evenings and save you some cash.

These days, society as a whole is *really* into soap — the cleaner the better! As little kids, we're told to scrub, scrub, scrub with plenty of soap and water. As teenagers, we use more soap — to fight acne and oily skin. As adults, we tend to follow the same routines even though our skin has changed. And the range of different types of soaps available is mind boggling — super-fatted, deodorant, rejuvenating, oatmeal, avocado, citrus, aloe vera, sandalwood, wintergreen, peppermint, patchouli, and vitamin E to name a few.

Many types of cleansers are also available. Some exfoliate as they clean, and the medicated ones generally contain benzoyl peroxide or salicylic acid in various concentrations. Overcleansing with these products can be irritating. More often than not, these items will only dry out and irritate your skin, particularly if you're already applying a topical anti-acne medication (see Chapters 7 and 9).

Washing excessively — more than twice a day — with any soap (regular soaps, acne soaps, antibacterial soaps, soaps with abrasives, or even gentle soaps) has little positive impact on your acne. In fact, if you have acne, your skin may be red and inflamed, and frequent washing only makes it redder.

Washing your face with a mild soap just twice a day is the best tactic, regardless of your skin type or acne activity. I recommend the following soaps and cleansers, depending on your skin type. These tried-and-true recommendations may not sound as exciting as a Provencal honey-lavender soap with grape seeds, but they flat out work:

- ✔ **Oily skin:** Ivory soap

- ✔ **Dry skin:** Dove soap

- ✔ **Extra-sensitive skin or allergic reaction to soaps:** Nonsoap cleanser such as Cetaphil, Aquanil, or Neutrogena Extra Gentle Cleanser

At the risk of sounding like a parent — with the whole "wash behind your ears" thing — now that you have your soap, here's how to use it:

1. **Get the soap wet, using lukewarm water.**

2. **Using your fingertips or a soft washcloth, apply the soap to your skin and rub it gently into your skin using a circular motion.** Don't use loofah sponges, brushes, or sandpaper please.

3. **Splash your face with lukewarm water until the soap is completely gone.** Expect to rinse your face for just a few seconds — perhaps as long as it would take to sing "Happy Birthday."

4. **Pat — don't rub — your skin until it's dry.** Use a soft cotton towel.

And that's it!

Dealing with dry skin

If you have overly dry skin (known as *xerosis* in the medical world), it's probably more of a problem for you when the weather is cold and the humidity is low. This occurs most often in the winter months in northern climates. In Western societies, our modern lifestyles also emphasize overbathing, which only serves to worsen the dryness. On top of that, we often live and work in overheated spaces.

If your skin is dry, keep it moist by using only mild soaps or soap substitutes as I recommend in the preceding section. You could also consider moving to a more humid climate — think rain forest. If you're already using a mild soap (and assuming a move to the Amazon is out of the question), apply moisturizers regularly, particularly *when your skin is still damp* (check out the "Giving your skin a drink!" sidebar in this chapter to find out why). Finding the right moisturizer for your skin may involve trial and error. Look for those that are labeled as noncomedogenic. I happen to recommend Oil of Olay, but many other excellent products are available. Go ahead and use a moisturizer that contains a sunscreen if you think you need one. You can also use room humidifiers to help hydrate your skin.

If you have acne and dry skin, you probably know that acne treatments can make your dry skin worse. Using moisturizers over your topical acne medicine can make these symptoms more tolerable. If you wear makeup, you can apply it over the moisturizer.

Some common recommendations for dry skin are of questionable or no value, including the following:

- ✔ Ingesting copious amounts of water
- ✔ Taking lots of vitamins

These "remedies" won't hurt you, but don't look to them to cure your dry skin. Instead, treat your acne and dry skin with TLC and the gentlest of cleansing methods.

If your skin gets flaky and scaly, that doesn't mean that you have wrinkles. In fact, several of the topical treatments that I cover in Chapter 9 can cause your skin to look dry and scaly as a side effect, but some of these medications can actually prevent wrinkles.

Coping with an oil glut

If you have excessively oily skin, that's due to your sebaceous glands producing more sebum (the acne-related oil that I discuss in detail in Chapter 3) than you'd like them to. This is often the case if you also happen to have acne. But for now, here are some tips on caring for your oily skin:

- ✔ Be happy that you'll save a few bucks on not buying moisturizers.

- ✔ Be happier because your skin will tend to stay more wrinkle-free and younger looking!

- ✔ Be even happier because your skin will tend to be less sensitive!

But you probably want some more concrete tips, so here you go:

- ✔ Even though your skin's oily, don't irritate it. Washing your face twice a day should be enough. I realize that you may have been told to wash 77 times a day with strong abrasive soaps, but that will only irritate your skin and make it redder — and if you have acne, all that scrubbing will only make it look worse! For advice on exactly how to wash your skin, check out "How to wash your face."

- ✔ If parts of your face feel oily during the day, the oil can be wiped away with a mild alcohol-and-water astringent such as Neutrogena Clear Pore Oil-Controlling Astringent, Noxzema Triple Clean Astringent, or Clean & Clear Advanced Acne Pads.

Giving your skin a drink!

The next time you take a long bath or stay in a swimming pool for a long time, notice how soggy and rippled the skin on your palms and soles looks after a while. That's because they've been immersed in water for a long period and your waterproof protective layer of *sebum* (the oily stuff that plays a large role in acne, as I discuss in Chapter 3) got washed away, so water can now get readily absorbed into the outer layer of your epidermis.

The rippling or wrinkled appearance develops because your skin has increased its surface area to accommodate all the water it absorbed during that time. It's water-logged! The "wrinkling" is so obvious on your palms and soles because they have the thickest stratum corneum. If you watch your hand for 5 minutes or so, you'll see that the corrugated look disappears. That's because the water soon evaporates from your overhydrated stratum corneum.

Now, if you apply a moisturizer before the water evaporates, you can "lock in" the water that was absorbed while you were bathing or showering. Moisturizers don't add water to the skin; instead, they reduce water loss by slowing its evaporation.

Your take home message: If you have dry skin, apply a moisturizer while your skin is still damp.

Chapter 3

Tracing the Evolution of a Pimple

Ah, the pimple. It's the bane of many a school picture and wedding day. Pimples help keep photo retouchers in business. But for many people, pimples aren't simple nuisances that pop up at inopportune times. Instead, they're a daily reminder that seemingly uncontrollable forces are at work in the skin.

In this chapter, I outline the events that are required to make acne lesions. (A *lesion* is dermatologist lingo for any abnormality or mark of the skin. A pimple is a lesion. A blackhead is a lesion. Your nose isn't a lesion, unless you have two of them.) I take you through many of the conditions necessary for a lesion to form and evolve: blocked hair follicles, overworked oil glands, and bacteria. Then I help you categorize your acne in order to understand when and why different treatments are used on the various types.

Paying the High Price for Oil

Acne lesions originate and mature in the hair follicle, the epicenter of our acne story. (To get a visual of what a normal, healthy follicle doing its job looks like, take a peek at Figure 3-1.) Ultimately, in order for acne to develop, a follicle must be blocked. A blocked follicle isn't the only condition necessary for acne to form (I detail the others in the sections that follow), but it's a big one. So, to talk about the roots of acne, you need to go directly to the hair follicle.

 Technically, the hair follicle and sebaceous gland are called the *pilosebaceous unit* (PSU). For simplicity sake, I just refer to the whole thing as the "follicle" or "hair follicle" in this book.

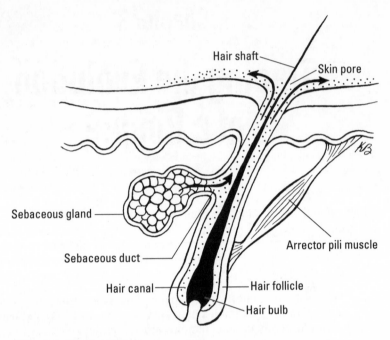

Figure 3-1: A normal follicle.

The hair follicle (actually the PSU) is made up of three components:

✔ **Sebaceous gland:** This gland resembles a cluster of grapes and produces and pumps out a beneficial oily substance called *sebum* (pronounced *see*-bum) that coats and conditions the hair and skin. The oily sebum is composed of a rich blend of different *lipids* (fatty chemicals). Sebum rises to the surface of your epidermis to keep your skin lubricated and protected. It also helps makes your skin waterproof. Plus, sebum helps carry dead skin cells out of the hair follicle and to the exterior skin so that the body can get rid of them.

In people with acne, there is an excessive production of sebum. Along with its producer, the sebaceous gland, its fellow cast member, the hair follicle, and its director *testosterone* (an important hormone), sebum plays much more than a bit part in the acne story.

✔ **Sebaceous duct:** This tiny tube steers the sebum (and the dead skin cells it carries) from the sebaceous gland into the *hair canal,* the part of the follicle through which sebum travels onto the hairs before it is carried out to the exterior of your skin.

✔ **Hair:** I'm talking about the actual hair that sprouts out of your pores (*follicular orifices,* or the holes in your skin that your hair grows out of). Hairs are sometimes called *strands* or *hair shafts*. Hairs are found all over our bodies; well, almost all over. There's no hair on your palms, I hope. Hairs help carry sebum to our skin.

Priming the pump with hormones

Hormones play a central role in the acne drama. *Hormones* are the body's chemical messengers. Without hormones, you wouldn't have acne, but you'd be in pretty bad shape, because hormones control just about every bodily function, from regulating your metabolism to ensuring that you can mature and have children.

In both males and females, a particular group of hormones, called *androgens,* are primarily associated with the formation of acne. The term *androgen* is a general term for hormones that have more masculinizing features. Androgens are responsible for the development of secondary sex characteristics in males (facial hair, increased muscle mass, the ability to reproduce, and so on). The androgen *testosterone* is the main male hormone. However, if you're female, you have androgens too, but they're produced in smaller quantities and are much weaker than in your male counterparts.

Estrogen and *progesterone* are the primary female hormones that control menstrual cycles and regulate pregnancy. Both of these hormones can have an affect on acne as well — albeit less than androgens — by their periodic monthly fluctuations. (I talk more about these hormones in Chapter 5.)

The androgenic hormones help us regulate how much sebum (the healthy oil I describe in the preceding section) our sebaceous glands produce. People who get acne aren't producing any more of these androgens than anyone else; it's just that their sebaceous glands are very sensitive to the hormone's message to increase production. The glands respond by pumping out excessive amounts of sebum. Your face, chest, and back contain the highest concentrations of sebaceous glands; that's why you're more likely to have acne on these areas.

Adolescence is generally the worst time for acne because androgens are increasing steadily during the teen years, and they signal your sebaceous glands to get larger and to generate more sebum, as shown in Figure 3-2. As adolescence ends, the amount of androgen secretion diminishes and acne tends to disappear for most teens by age 18 or 19. But for various reasons that I discuss in Chapter 5, some women (and much less commonly, men) retain a heightened sensitivity to their androgens and continue to have acne beyond adolescence. Some women even get acne for the first time as adults.

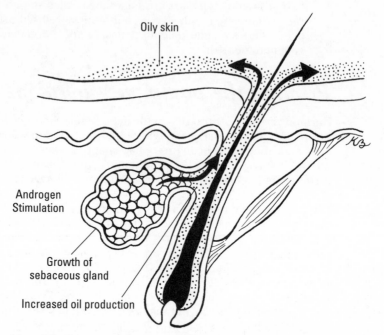

Figure 3-2: The sebaceous gland overreacts to androgen stimulation.

Clogging your pores and narrowing the hair canal

Every day, millions of skin cells die off. You continually make new skin cells and get rid of dead ones. Your body has ingenious ways of getting rid of these dead cells. In the case of your skin, sebum carries the dead skin cells to the outside of the body where they flake off.

Sometimes, though, as sebum ferries dead cells from the inside of your hair follicle along the oily sebaceous ducts and out through the hair canal, the exit route of the follicle is blocked by the excess oil. This blockage causes the opening of your hair canal to narrow, and your *pores,* the tiny openings in your skin that serve as exits for your hairs, get clogged (see Figure 3-3). The exit of oil is also often impeded by a process called *abnormal follicular keratinization.* That's a fancy way of saying that instead of flaking off with the sebum when they reach the skin's surface as they normally do, the dead skin cells and keratin clump together with the oil to further clog the sebaceous ducts and hair canals.

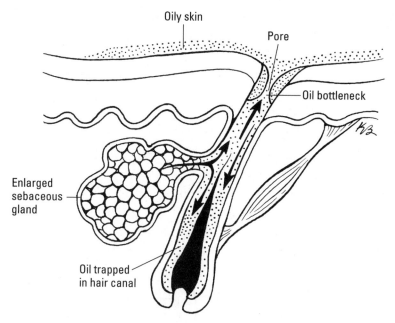

Figure 3-3: The clogging of pores and the narrowing of the hair canal.

Acne is *not* caused by forgetting to wash the oil off, or even by eating loads of greasy French fries and junk food. It's not the oil in your tummy or *on* your skin; it's the oil *in* your skin.

Forming blackheads and whiteheads

The trapped sebum, cells, and keratin form a very sticky mixture — a real traffic jam that blocks the exit route. This plug acts just like a cork in a bottle, locking in all that stuff inside with nowhere to go, so that it can't exit onto the surface of the skin (see Figure 3-4). The plug is called a *microcomedo* (pronounced *my*-kro-*cahm*-e-doe). You can't see a microcomedo with the naked eye; it's too small. Over time, the increasing amount of trapped sebum builds up a lot of pressure and the hair follicle blows up like a balloon and becomes a visible *comedo* (pronounced *cahm*-e-doe; the plural of comedo is *comedones*).

There are the two types of comedones (which you can see in Figure 3-4 and also in the color section of this book):

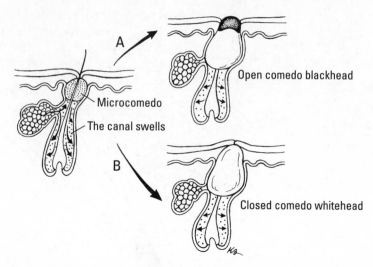

Figure 3-4: The microcomedo forms and becomes either a blackhead (A) or a whitehead (B).

- **Blackheads:** If the comedo enlarges and pops out through the surface of the skin, the tip looks dark and it's called a blackhead. The dark color is *not due to dirt;* it's the result of a buildup of *melanin,* a dark pigment in the skin that turns black when exposed to oxygen in the air. Blackheads are also known as *open comedones.*

- **Whiteheads:** If the comedo stays below the surface of the skin, it's light in color and looks like a small whitish bump; it's called a whitehead. Whiteheads are also called *closed comedones.*

Comedogenesis is the medical term for the process that forms whitehead and blackheads.

Battling bacteria

The microcomedo may develop into, and remain, a comedo. But sometimes it becomes an inflammatory lesion. *Inflammation* is a reaction of the skin to disease or injury; in the case of acne, the inflammation is a reaction to the bacteria known as *Propionibacterium acnes.* Signs of an inflammatory lesion include swelling, redness, heat, and sometimes pain. The presence of these bacteria does not mean that poor hygiene is a cause of your acne.

Here's a list of common inflammatory acne lesions:

✔ **Papule:** A small, firm red bump, commonly referred to as a pimple or zit. It's made up of inflammatory blood cells and doesn't contain obvious pus.

✔ **Pustule:** A papule that contains pus, a whitish, goopy substance that's really just a bunch of white blood cells. Pustules are also known as "pus pimples."

✔ **Nodule:** A large and often tender, lumpy, inflamed, pus-filled papule or pustule that's lodged more deeply in the skin. The term *cyst* is often used interchangeably to mean "nodule" because of the resemblance of a nodular acne lesion to a cyst.

One other common acne lesion is sometimes formed late in the life cycle of a lesion from the remains of an inflammatory lesion:

✔ **Macule:** A macule is a flat red, purple, or brown spot that forms where a papule or pustule used to be. A macule remains for a while after an acne lesion has healed or is in the process of healing. For more details on how your skin heals, check out Chapter 16.

To see what the preceding lesions look like, take a look at the color section of this book.

P. acnes jumps in

In order for comedones to move up the inflammation chain into a full-blown lesion, they need the help of a certain bacteria. You know how people add yeast to make a cake rise? Well, the bacterium known as *Propionibacterium acnes* helps make the zits rise. From now on, I just call him (or is it her?) *P. acnes,* for short.

P. acnes is an *anaerobe*. That means that it prefers to live in areas that have very little oxygen such as in the low oxygen environment that exists in a hair follicle.

P. acnes generally minds its own business. These usually "friendly" and harmless bacteria are present on everybody's skin, but in the proper environment (like a nice roomy, oily, hair follicle), they can cause trouble: In some kids and adults who are predisposed to have acne, *P. acnes* invade the plugged hair follicles (the comedones) and multiply.

These *P. acnes* never become bored or go hungry because they continuously munch on the oily, fatty sebum that serves as a food supply for them. They accomplish this culinary feat by producing chemicals known as enzymes. *Enzymes* are proteins that cause a chemical change in other substances without being changed themselves. *P. acnes* enzymes are like our knives and forks that help us to chop up our food into smaller pieces so that it's digestible.

It's Latin to me

The word *comedo* means a "glutton" in Latin and derives from a verb meaning to eat. I guess the microcomedo must be a little glutton? The word is *comer* to those of you who know some Spanish. Do you think the ancient Romans knew about the voracious eating habits of *P. acnes,* or did they just think that acne was caused by eating too much Roman junk food? Another conjecture has it that the ancients imagined the blackhead to be a flesh-eating maggot or "flesh worm." Gross!

The *P. acnes* produces the enzyme *lipase,* which can split apart certain fats (triglicerides) into smaller pieces (free fatty acids) so they can digest them.

P. acnes eating breakfast, lunch, and dinner, combined with the force of the trapped sebum, can cause ruptures or leaks in the wall of the comedo, allowing the free fatty acids into the surrounding dermis. (Check out Chapter 2 for information about the dermis, the skin layer that's below your epidermis.)

Calling all white blood cells!

When the bacteria start to use their lipases to produce free fatty acids, this causes other chemical 911 signals to be sent to your white blood cells. That's because the free fatty acids are very irritating to the skin. Your body responds to the irritation by recruiting an army of red and white blood cells (sounds like the Russian revolution!) to seal off the area where the free fatty acids and bacteria are located. White blood cells are your body's natural defense system. They rush to the scene accompanied by red blood cells to try to clean up the mess. Despite their good intentions, sometimes these helpful little cells overdo it and produce inflammatory acne lesions. The cleanup attempt results in red, swollen pimples or pustules that may even lead to even larger lumps, papules, and nodules. See Figure 3-5.

Scarring: Your skin's repair kit

The responsibility of repairing any injury that takes place belongs to cells in the dermis known as *fibroblasts.* These cells produce collagen. The collagen in your dermis plays the major role in patching up any damage to your skin. When there is an overproduction of collagen, the excess collagen becomes piled up in fibrous masses, resulting in a characteristic firm scar. The *P. acnes* bacterium can also contribute to destruction by releasing tissue-destroying chemicals that can damage normal collagen, and result in scarring.

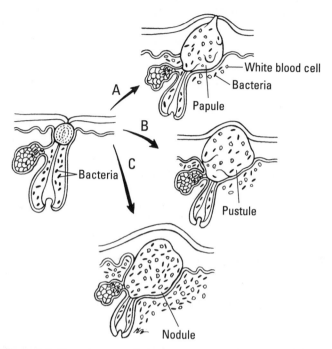

Figure 3-5: The microcomedo becomes an inflammatory papule (A), pustule (B), or nodule (C).

Acne scars are the visible reminders of where the body's inflammatory battle against an acne lesion took place. The deeper an acne lesion is lodged in the skin, the greater the chance for scarring. For more on scars and healing, take a gander at Chapter 16.

Classifying Acne

It's important for us dermatologists to be able to describe acne in various categories. It helps us to better understand what our patients have to say and it helps us to communicate with one another. It also helps us to follow the progress or lack of progress in our treatments. Here are the basic categories of acne; terms that you'll run into later in this book, and likely in your doctor's office:

  ✔ **Non-inflammatory acne:** This category of acne is identified when a person's lesions are primarily whiteheads and blackheads. It's sometimes called *comedonal acne,* because it's characterized by comedones.

✔ **Inflammatory acne:** In this type of acne, papules or pustules, red or purple macules, and nodules, often termed "cysts," are predominant.

A single patient can have a combination of both non-inflammatory and inflammatory acne. Typically, this combination is seen in teenagers rather than adults. Adults more often have inflammatory acne. The way acne is treated often depends on which type you have:

✔ For acne that is primarily comedonal with blackheads and whiteheads, we use agents known as retinoids, such as Retin-A, Differin, or Tazorac to treat them. These drugs are comedolytic, which means they break up comedones.

✔ If you have inflammatory acne, we tend to rely more often on benzoyl peroxide and/or topical and oral antibiotics.

✔ If you have a combination of both types of acne, we tend to use benzoyl peroxide in combination with the retinoids.

You can read more about these treatments, and many others, in Part III.

A mountain or a molehill?

Keep in mind that one person's "mild" is another person's "severe" and vice versa: To illustrate this point, I must tell you about two types of patients:

A 35-year-old man appeared in my office covered with papules, pustules, nodules, and scars on his face and chest. When I asked him for the reason for his visit, he pointed to his finger and said, "For this wart."

He wasn't in the least concerned about what I considered to be his severe acne. I couldn't resist, so I asked him about it and he said, "All the men in my family have acne and I, like them, have no problem living with it. I'm married, and my wife couldn't care less about it either," he continued. So I treated his wart and he left with a smile.

On the other hand, I have several patients, both male and female, who call me every few months, feeling extremely upset if they get even one small pimple on their chins. Go figure!

Moral: A pimple is in the eyes of the beholder, or one person's mountain is another person's molehill.

Part II
Figuring Out Your Acne and How to Tackle It on Your Own

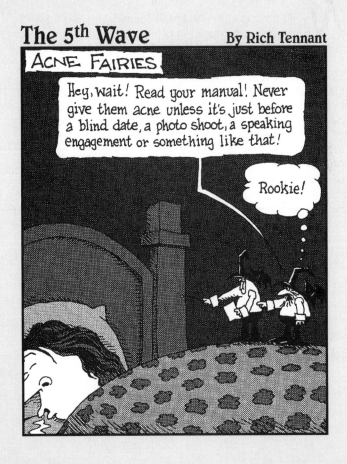

In this part . . .

*N*ot all acne is alike. Acne has many faces and features, and the condition often varies according to age group (teens and adults) and gender. So, I spend some time in this part distinguishing between the signs and symptoms of teenage acne, which affects both boys and girls, and adult-onset acne, which largely targets females in their 20s, 30s, and beyond. I also set the record straight by weighing in on the various factors that some people claim make your acne worse. Finally, I provide you with a complete guide to over-the-counter acne-fighting preparations, explaining how to use them, what to expect, and what side effects to be on the lookout for.

Chapter 4

Examining Acne in Teens

. . . .

. . . .

*A*cne is the most common skin problem that teenagers face. Just about nine out of ten of them have to deal with pimples or acne at some time. That's right, nearly 90 percent of kids have to deal with at least an occasional breakout of pimples.

In this chapter, I give you the lowdown on teenage acne. I help you spot teenage acne in all its glory. I help you deal with the emotional scars of acne. And I remind you (or tell you for the first time if you haven't heard it before) that you don't have to accept acne as a rite of passage. You can do something about it.

Identifying Teenage Acne

We dermatologists generally refer to the acne that you get as a teenager as *acne vulgaris*. Yeah, it sounds horrible, but *vulgaris* is the Latin word for "common," not "obnoxious" or "repugnant." And as you saw in the stats I just tossed around, *common* is a good choice of words! (Some adults also suffer from acne vulgaris that sticks around after the teen years turn to the 20s and beyond. But most adults usually have a somewhat different type of acne, which I discuss in Chapter 5.)

In teenagers, acne is one of the signals that your body is going through a tremendous upheaval called puberty (see the "Understanding the Causes of Teenage Acne" section, later in the chapter, for details). Teenage acne often begins around the ages of

10 to 13. It may start before puberty in both sexes, but teenage girls tend to start getting acne at a younger age than boys; however, boys tend to have the more severe cases.

Studies have shown that puberty is occurring at an earlier age these days, and so is acne. Most teenagers grow out of it when they reach 19 or 20; however, don't be surprised if your acne persists into your early 20s and even into later adulthood.

But just because acne is common and almost every teen suffers through it doesn't mean you can't do anything about it. You don't have to just wait for it to go away. That's what I'm here for — to help you knock out those pimples, whiteheads, and blackheads. With so many excellent acne treatments available today, treating your acne will prevent (or at least greatly lessen) the scarring that often results from untreated acne.

The curious case of the mail-order miracle

Jonathan is 16. He first started getting acne when he was about 14 when he saw a few small whiteheads and blackheads on his forehead and nose. Then his skin became greasy. His mom told him that if he just washed his face more often, his skin would look better and the pimples would clear up. But despite increased washing, his acne got worse and he started developing a few red pimples in addition to the whiteheads and blackheads. His mom started buying an acne cream from the drugstore. Jonathan tried it for a few months and it seemed to help a little.

But when he turned 16, he became really embarrassed and extremely self-conscious about how bad his acne made him look and he hated going to school. His mom then ordered a product that she saw advertised by doctors and movie stars on television. It was very expensive, but it promised to stop Jonathan's acne in its tracks! So Mom began ordering it by mail on a monthly basis. But just like the other over-the-counter product that she tried, this one helped a little, but not for long.

By the time his mother brought him to me, Jonathan's acne was completely out of control, and the mail-order product was starting to really irritate his face. After a few months of prescription cream medication, his face became almost completely free of acne! I reminded Jonathan and his mom about a few key points: You can't wash acne away, and in many cases washing your face too frequently or scrubbing too hard can worsen the appearance of acne (see Chapter 2). I also mentioned that it's hard for movie stars and "television doctors" who have never even seen your skin to make the correct diagnosis, let alone know exactly the best way to treat *your* personal skin problem.

Not that many teens have real problems (like scars or serious emotional problems) from acne, but if you do, there are a bunch of things that can be done to help you with those issues as well. In Chapters 16 and 17, I cover the physical scars and the emotional ride that some teens with acne have to endure.

If you want to jump ahead, you can check out Part III, where I provide advice on tackling the problem with the help of a dermatologist. Or take a look at Chapter 7, where I have advice on how to handle it on your own. Read on, though, if you want the full story on teen skin and the acne that it hosts. (You can also check out the sidebars throughout this and other chapters for stories about some of my real patients.)

Taking a look at teen skin

Teenagers' faces are all different. Your skin may be dark or light complexioned. You may have dry skin, oily skin, combination skin, sensitive skin, or be "thick-skinned" (I'm talking blowtorch-resistant, here). I can't generalize, but there are a couple of tendencies that make your skin different from that of adults:

- ✔ **More oiliness and less sensitivity:** Teen skin tends to be a little oilier, and that's probably a good thing because many treatments that are effective for teenage acne can be somewhat irritating to the more sensitive skin that commonly affects adults. The extra oil serves as a waterproof barrier between you and the outside world and protects your skin from irritation. In Chapters 7, 9, and 10, I list some of the different medications that can be used to treat acne-prone skin.

- ✔ **Easier to heal:** Your skin tends to be more "forgiving" and to heal more completely after experiencing acne. This is especially important when it comes to avoiding permanent scars and those dark spots that tend to appear in people of color when their acne lesions heal. I go into physical scars of acne in Chapter 16 and the dark spots and other issues related to acne in dark complexioned skin in Chapter 12.

Exploring teen acne

Good ol' acne vulgaris, teenage acne. If you have it, you have an idea what it looks like (or you can take a look at the color section of this book for a photo). But there may be more in store. Plus, if you skipped over Chapter 3, getting a handle on some of the terminology here can help you out if your dermatologist starts throwing it around. So, without further delay, here are the main features of teen acne:

✔ **Centered on the T-zone:** Typically, teenage acne tends to flare up on the forehead, nose, and chin. Take a look at Figure 4-1 to see a picture of this T-zone. Sometimes however, acne can have a mind of its own and it can pop up anywhere on your face or trunk.

✔ **Blackheads and whiteheads:** We dermatologists call these two unwelcome visitors *comedones*. Actually we call black-heads *open comedones* and whiteheads *closed comedones*. (You have to turn to Chapter 3 to find out why, though.) These black and white bumps are largely the upshot of teen acne and aren't so common in adults.

✔ **Inflammatory lesions:** These acne lesions are called papules, pustules, nodules, and cysts. These are the red, pus-filled, lumpy, inflamed, and sometimes sore, painful zits.

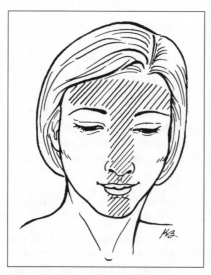

Figure 4-1: Teens often experience acne flare ups in the T-zone.

Tracking acne's footsteps

In its full glory, teenage acne generally looks like a mixture of blackheads and whiteheads (comedonal acne) with papules and pustules (inflammatory acne) and macules (healing lesions). Awesome! Here's how teenage acne can look in different kids. Maybe you'll find your type in one of the following descriptions:

✔ Initially, the main lesions may be whiteheads and blackheads. Often they start out in a nice, embarrassing, central location — the nose and forehead. This part of the T-zone is where your skin tends to be most oily and, therefore, likely to develop acne.

As time goes on, you may discover a zit (also called pimples or papules; the red stuff) here and there, and an additional blackhead or whitehead now and then. There's a good chance that they will come and go. At this point, we're still in the "it's no big thing" stage. This type of acne is a rite of passage that almost all of us go through. If you're lucky, this will just pass by itself or you can help it clear up with some inexpensive over-the-counter stuff that you can buy at your local drug-store (see Chapter 7 for the names of these medications).

✔ Sometimes, however, the going can get a little rougher: The whiteheads and blackheads want to hang around a lot longer and sometimes a population spurt of inflammatory papules and pustules really start making their presence felt. They can be seen in the center of the face but may also be scattered all over the place including your neck, chest, and back.

If you have dark skin, you may not see all of this red stuff because your acne may look brown or even darker on your skin (see Chapter 12 where I go into acne that's seen in darker skin).

As individual acne lesions heal, *macules* (dark red or purple spots) form and linger until the lesion heals completely. The macules may look brown or almost black in color if you are very dark-complexioned.

✔ In some teens, especially those who have inherited a tendency to develop scarring acne, acne nodules may appear. They can get quite large, lumpy, and painful. They're inflamed lesions that are situated deeper than ordinary papules and pustules and can, if they go untreated, leave deep or thickened scars. This is called nodular acne (see Chapter 3 for a full description).

Fortunately, even if acne reaches this point, dermatologists can treat it very effectively in many people with oral antibiotics and, if necessary, with an oral retinoid, known as isotretinoin, or Accutane. (I discuss this powerful drug in Chapter 13.) Besides these strong medicines, we have many new tricks up our sleeves, such as lasers and special lights to treat your acne. Chapters 14 and 16 explain these cutting-edge treatments.

It's Greek to me

The original name for acne was derived from the Greek word akm — and Latin acme meaning high point or peak. I'm thinking the name came from the fact that some of the pimples looked like the size of Mount Olympus to akm — sufferers.

Understanding the Causes of Teenage Acne

You may think you have teenage acne as some sort of punishment for a crime you didn't even know you committed. Actually though, you're breaking out for two main reasons. The first is that, as you mature, your hormones are telling your oil glands to produce too much oil, and your body isn't handling the oil very well. Another reason you're breaking out? Well, you may be able to go ahead and blame your parents or other ancestors for this one. Heredity plays a huge role in whether you end up with acne. In this section, I go over both topics to give you a better idea of why you're breaking out. (In Chapter 6, I provide you with many other theories and possible causes of acne.)

Passing through puberty: Hormones gone wild

By the time you hit puberty, it may seem like all you hear about is hormones and how they're to blame for every problem you have, from shyness to a low paying job to acne. In the case of acne, what people are telling you is the truth. Hormones *are* to blame!

Hormones are the chemical messengers that provide the signals that regulate many of your body's functions and that are responsible for the changes you experience during puberty. They're also responsible for bringing your acne to the forefront. (I go into more detail on hormones in Chapter 3.)

 The most important hormones when it comes to acne are your androgens. *Androgens* are really a group of closely related hormones. The androgen *testosterone* is the main "male" hormone. Besides bringing on puberty-related changes, it's also central to our acne story.

Androgens are a natural part of development for both boys and girls, but boys tend to produce more of them, especially testosterone, which is why boys have bigger bodies and stubbly beards. The higher level of testosterone in boys is considered to be the reason that they tend to get more severe breakouts of acne than do girls. As in males, androgens also are necessary for the development of acne in females.

Estrogen and *progesterone* are female hormones that play the primary role in puberty. These female hormones play less important roles in the evolution of teenage acne than do androgens, but their influence on acne's ups and downs, as well as their part in its treatment, is significant. I talk about both of them in relation to adult-onset acne in Chapter 5, and I tell how they're used in the treatment of acne in Chapter 10.

Dousing occasional flare-ups

When she was in eighth grade, Margot's parents had taken her to see a dermatologist who prescribed a cream and a gel. This approach worked very well for several years and kept her acne under good control. However, during midterms in her sophomore year of college, she began getting red bumps all over her face. She started to wear a coverup makeup, which she hated to use. "It looked so artificial," she said. "I stopped going out on dates; I was so embarrassed about the way I looked." Moreover, her pimples would flare up "like clockwork" right before her periods.

When I first saw her in my office, I recommended that *oral antibiotics* (acne medications that are taken by mouth) might help to clear up her skin. She said that she was somewhat reluctant to start taking them because she was concerned about the possible dangers, but nonetheless agreed to start taking them.

On a subsequent appointment, she was very pleased with how much progress she'd made. Her face was looking better and her red pimples were now flat, so she could more easily cover them with makeup. I then suggested that she gradually taper off the oral antibiotic by lowering her dosage and suggested that hopefully she could "wean" herself off of the oral therapy and see if the cream and gel alone would do the job. If not, I told her that we could try the oral method again, if necessary.

The system worked very well. Except for breakouts before her period, Margot's acne was not much of a problem. On several occasions during her junior and senior years, she required the oral antibiotics and they continued to have success in quelling her bad flare-ups.

During puberty, the levels of androgens in both boys and girls starts to climb and begins to stimulate your oil glands to grow and produce more sebum. If you develop acne, you probably don't have higher amounts of these androgens; it's more likely that you have a higher sensitivity to them. You can flip back to Chapter 3 to see how this happens.

And how's this for an entry in the "perfect timing" category: Just when you guys begin to shave, up pop those bumps that get in the way of your razor. Now you have the added problem of having to shave over and around those papules and pustules. It's like an obstacle course! Turn to Chapter 19 where I give some shaving advice.

Thanking your family: The heredity factor

That's right. You may be able to thank your mom, dad, aunts, uncles, and grandparents for the current state of your face. Check in with your parents and their siblings to see whether they've had acne too and how severe it was. If acne runs in your family (or even hides — it may be lurking under shirts and blouses!), you're more likely to have it too. Feel free to drop them a thank-you note.

If both of your parents had acne, you're even more likely to have it. In fact, identical twins tend to share acne problems just like they share looks. And they got their acne genes from their parents, who inherited them from their parents, and so on, probably back to the Stone Age.

Why is acne hereditary? Well, for the same reason anything is inherited from your parents: for instance, the color of your skin, eyes, and hair. Scientists are still trying to pinpoint the exact genetic cause or causes of acne. We do know that you inherited *something* from your parents that tells your body:

- ✔ How much oil to produce

- ✔ How big or small your oil glands are

- ✔ How sensitive your oil glands are to androgens

- ✔ How easily your pores get clogged

- ✔ How quickly your skin cells replace themselves

- ✔ How quickly your immune system reacts to the acne-producing bacteria, *P. acnes.*

All these instructions are just swimming in your gene pool. And sometimes, what finally emerges is often just a matter of luck! For more on how these points meld together to actually form acne, turn to Chapter 3.

If you were adopted, you inherited the acne tendency from your biological family.

Acknowledging the Emotional

Acne can be difficult to deal with at any age. But for teens, the appearance of acne can be especially trying. Who has time to deal with this stuff? At a time in your life when you're working on your homework, social life, dating, trying out for the school play, and getting a job (among all the other activities and events in life), developing acne can seem like a major bump in the road. You've got better things to do with your time. But there's a lot that you can do to control acne without letting your life get out of control.

Maybe you feel totally alone. Maybe you just want to stay in your room, pull the covers over your head, curl up into a little ball, and hide away forever. Maybe you feel worthless and you want to give up. Guess what! I don't think I've ever met a teenager — even those without acne — who doesn't feel that way at some time or other. It's natural! Even adults get that way sometimes.

You may feel uncomfortable talking about acne. Acne can be embarrassing, but I'm sure there are people to talk to if you give it a shot. If you try talking to trusted friends, your doctor, or your parents or other family members, I think you'll be surprised by how helpful they are!

Close to 90 percent of teens face acne at some point in their lives, which means that 90 percent of adults also know how it feels. For more on dealing with the emotional side of acne, and getting out of those emotional ruts that accompany it, see Chapter 17.

Chapter 5

Addressing Acne in Adults

· ·

· ·

*H*igh school is a memory. You have a career, you're going to college, or you're raising a family. You've settled down. Acne, you assume, is a thing of the past. But just when you think that you're out of the woods, acne hits you right in the face.

Dermatologists regularly hear the lament "Acne, at my age?!" expressed by women who suddenly develop acne after the ages of 20 or 30. "It's not fair; it's supposed to be only for teenagers!" is usually the next statement out of their mouths. It may not be fair, but it's a fact. Many people — mostly women — get acne for the first time as adults or develop acne after years of being relatively pimple free. And sometimes teenage acne can continue unabated from teen years into adulthood.

In this chapter, I prepare you for some surprising occasions when acne can rear its ugly head — adulthood, pregnancy, and menopause. Adult-onset acne is overwhelmingly a condition seen in women. Therefore, I spend the bulk of this chapter discussing adult-onset acne as it relates to women. And as always, I show you that there is hope to help your acne symptoms clear up. But if you're one of the relatively few guys facing acne as an adult, don't worry; I help you get a handle on your condition at the end of the chapter.

Identifying Adult-Onset Acne

Adult-onset acne is a type of acne that turns up after the age of 18 — somewhat later than the typical teenage variety of acne. It can crop up during a woman's 20s, 30s, or even later in life. Adult-onset acne, sometimes referred to as *female adult acne* or *post-adolescent acne*, is overwhelmingly a condition of females.

The fluctuating nature of adult-onset acne tends to make the influence of hormones more obvious than with the typical case of teenage acne vulgaris (see Chapter 4); however, teenage girls often begin to note those premenstrual pimply "ups" and "downs" as they approach adulthood. As many woman are aware, the lesions have a propensity to come and go more readily than they do with teenage acne, and their appearance and disappearance is often linked to their menstrual cycle (see the "Acne and your menstrual cycle" section, later in the chapter).

Describing the symptoms

The appearance of post-adolescent acne differs from that of teenage acne:

- ✔ Blackheads and whiteheads (comedones) are less commonly seen.

- ✔ Breakouts are usually mild to moderate.

- ✔ Significant scarring is unusual (but the term "significant" is a relative and in the in eyes of the person who has acne, it can be *very* significant).

- ✔ Lesions more often appear on the lower cheek, the chin, and along and below the jaw line. Although some women may have breakouts on the chest and back, most have blemishes exclusively on the face.

Breakouts are usually limited to inflammatory papules (pimples, bumps, zits), pustules, and small inflammatory nodules. (Check out the color section of this book for the typical appearance of adult-onset acne.) The papules and pustules can be superficial or deep. Many women describe certain papules as "deep ones," the ones that feel like they come from under the skin. (If you get 'em, you know what I mean.) The deep ones are often more *palpable*

Checking under the hood

Emily, a 33-year-old stockbroker, came to my office. She told me that she had very mild acne as a teenager that cleared up by the time she was 19, but returned out of nowhere. Since then, she'd noticed increasing numbers of red pimples on her chin that tended to appear regularly a few days before her period and lasted only for a few days. Some of the bumps seemed to come from under her skin and many of these remained in place for a long time.

When I looked at her face, I noted that she had a few, very subtle reddish blotches on her chin, but otherwise had an almost perfectly clear complexion. Then she said, "Oh, you should have seen my face two weeks ago when I made this appointment! I can't believe it. It's just like when I brought my car in to have the auto mechanic check out a loud squealing noise and — of course — it didn't squeak or even squeal when he test drove it!"

Based upon her history, I concluded that she had typical adult-onset acne that has its ups and downs, and I just happened to be seeing her on an up day. I also suggested that she might need a new fan belt for her car.

I then prescribed a prescription gel for her to apply to her skin. I suggested that she apply it daily and I explained that it might help to break her adult-onset acne cycle. She scheduled a return appointment. As it turned out, she canceled the return visit, and several months later, she sent me the following note: "Thanks! My face is pretty clear now, but my car still squeals." I guess I'll stick with dermatology!

(you're able to feel, or *palpate* them) than visible. They represent papules and pustules that haven't reached, and may never reach, the surface of the skin.

When these deep lesions grow even larger, they're called nodules (or cysts). *Nodules* are tender, firm lumps that may hang around for weeks or months. They may grow to an inch or more in diameter and can leave scars after they heal. Fortunately, nodules and subsequent scarring are infrequently seen in women who have adult-onset acne. (In Chapter 3, you can find out more about nodules. In Chapter 16, I discuss scarring.)

The diagnosis of adult-onset acne isn't always clear-cut. Your healthcare provider may easily confuse adult-onset acne with other acnelike disorders:

  ✔ **Rosacea:** Symptoms of rosacea include facial lesions that consist of acnelike red papules and pustules. Moreover, both rosacea and acne can appear together. (I talk about how to distinguish between the two in Chapter 18.)

✔ **Pseudofolliculitis barbae and keratosis pilaris:** These conditions involve hair follicles, and can sometimes be acne look-alikes. (I cover these acne impostors in Chapter 19.)

✔ **Endocrinopathy:** Sometimes what appears to be a simple case of acne vulgaris or adult-onset acne can be due to an underlying hormonal abnormality, called endocrinopathy (pronounced en-de-krin-op-ath-ee). At times like this, acne may be difficult to get under control, and other measures such as blood tests to look for higher or lower than normal hormone levels should be evaluated by your doctor. (I discuss this relatively infrequent but serious situation in Chapter 20.)

Taking an emotional toll

Having acne can be just as trying for adults as it is for teens. Job hunting, social events, and dating can be negatively impacted by a few pimples. Even mild acne that might seem insignificant to an outsider can force some people to miss out on opportunities and relationships that otherwise they might have explored. I offer some advice for managing the psychological burdens of acne in Chapter 17. Whether you have rather mild or severe acne, effective treatments are available, and your condition can improve. Look at the sidebars in this chapter for stories about patients with varying degrees of acne. The patients discussed may have the same type of acne you have.

Emerging at Any Age

When acne begins in the teenage years, the increase in your androgens — male hormones that are present in both men and women — play a major role in its development. Chapter 3 explains this process, but in a nutshell, these hormones stimulate the sebaceous glands, enlarging them, and they respond by producing excessive oil that helps to promote the lesions of acne.

Although the entire story isn't well understood, the vast majority of women who have adult-onset acne don't have elevated androgen levels; rather, they appear to have an increased *response* to normal levels of androgen, and to a much lesser degree, to their female hormone, progesterone, that also has androgenic effects. The other major female hormone, estrogen, has an opposite (estrogenic) effect and tends to curb acne.

In addition to a woman's own hormones, adult-onset acne may be related to, and heightened by, the ingestion of external hormones and drugs that have androgenic effects such as those contained in certain oral contraceptive medications, food products, and performance enhancing drugs.

In the sections that follow, I outline common points in your life at which acne can be an issue and delve into why this may occur.

Acne and your menstrual cycle

If you're reading this, I probably don't have to tell you about those little red bumps that appear on a monthly basis. You're probably well aware of those unwelcome visitors that appear, disappear, and reappear like clockwork during your menstrual cycle. They usually last for several days, but sometimes they can persist for a month or longer. No fun!

When the going gets tough

Johanna, a teary-eyed, anxious, 23-year-old file clerk told me that she had suffered with acne "all" her life. After my usual comment that she must have been an unusual acne-covered baby at birth, she then told me that she had been suffering from acne since seventh grade (I guess that seemed like "forever" to her). As she held her head down, she said that she was ashamed to look at people and that when she was in high school some of the kids used to call her "pizza face."

And, indeed, her acne was severe. She had pimples, pustules, and nodules, as well as blackheads and whiteheads all over her face, shoulders, chest, and upper back. She told me that she had tried "everything," by which she meant numerous over-the-counter preparations that only served to irritate her skin but did little to get rid of the acne.

Her life was very limited and she stayed home most of the time because social situations made her very anxious and self-conscious. She felt that the few friends she had tended to avoid her. Her "best friend" advised her to wash her face more frequently. She felt dirty and embarrassed. She especially dreaded times when she would have to see her relatives at family holiday get-togethers. She preferred to interact with people over the telephone or by e-mail.

I saw Johanna in my office for several years. We used both topical and oral therapy to get her acne under reasonable control. She was left with some residual scars that I couldn't do too much about, but she seems to now relate more comfortably with people. And now at age 26 she has a new job as a medical secretary that is better paying, and yes, it keeps her in the public eye.

Most often, pimples tend to pop up right before your period. This is the time — usually two to seven days before your period — when estrogen levels fall and progesterone levels rise and stimulate the sebaceous glands to produce extra oil; with this extra oil comes acne.

Much less commonly, you may see no apparent connection between the appearance of pimples and your menstrual cycle. In such instances, they will erupt with a mind of their own only right before you have that important date, interview, cocktail party, public speaking engagement, or wedding! Great!!

New baby, new bumps: Acne and pregnancy

During pregnancy, acne is unpredictable. For some lucky women, the result is a welcome surprise — clear skin, the "glow of pregnancy" that you were told about. If this is your case, enjoy it! But don't get overconfident. When existing acne virtually disappears during pregnancy, it often recurs afterward — sorry!

However, existing acne can also get worse. Pregnancy is a time of tremendous hormonal upheaval. Your levels of estrogen and progesterone are rising, and your skin becomes more sensitive to the changes in the circulating hormones in your body. In fact, some women may experience acne for the first time when they become pregnant, even if they never had acne during their teens.

Acne is a perfectly normal occurrence during pregnancy (more common than most women realize), whether you have previously had acne or not. There's no way to prevent it from developing during pregnancy, but be patient and, with time, your skin will probably clear up and return to its natural, pre-pregnancy state.

Lesions during pregnancy are generally inflammatory in their appearance and typically take the form of papules, pustules, and sometimes nodules. (Check out Chapter 3 for information on different types of acne lesions.)

Acne tends to be worse during the first trimester (the first three months) of pregnancy when the levels of these hormones are increasing. Your progesterone is more androgenic (male hormone-like) than estrogen and causes the secretions of your skin glands to increase, which can lead to more acne. There are also times when your sebaceous glands go into high gear during the first, second, and third trimesters, causing even more frequent and serious breakouts.

When breastfeeding, some of the hormones that trigger your acne during pregnancy may still be at work, and you may wish to continues treating those pesky pimples. But be aware, as I mention in the sections that follow, that certain medications taken by mouth or applied to your skin may wind up in your breast milk.

Safe acne drugs when you're pregnant

The best course is to "say no" to any unnecessary drugs if you're pregnant or breastfeeding. Your baby is your first concern and you want to minimize any potentially harmful agents that might reach her. That said, the best way to treat acne during pregnancy is with a topical acne-fighting preparation. (Check out Chapters 9, 10, and 11 for details on the agents I mention in this section as well as other medications that fight acne.)

If you're planning to get pregnant, discuss your acne treatments with your dermatologist or healthcare provider. Some of the medications that are safely used to treat acne when you aren't pregnant may be potentially harmful to a developing fetus.

Topical treatments that your doctor may prescribe during pregnancy (and I discuss in Chapter 9) include:

- ✔ **Erythromycin:** There are many topical prescription products that contain this antibiotic.

- ✔ **Benzamycin Gel:** Benzamycin Gel combines erythromycin and benzoyl peroxide.

- ✔ **Azelaic acid:** This is a natural chemical produced by a yeast. It is the active ingredient in the prescription products Azelex and Finevin.

The U.S. Food and Drug Administration (FDA) classifies Azelaic acid as a pregnancy category B drug. This designation means that animal reproduction studies have failed to demonstrate a risk to the fetus; however, there are no adequate and well-controlled studies in pregnant humans.

Because passage of the drug into maternal milk may occur, this drug should be used during pregnancy or by nursing mothers only if clearly needed.

On the whole, I recommend that you avoid all oral medicines to treat acne when you're pregnant. However, oral erythromycin — if you're not allergic to it — may be taken safely if your acne is really bad. If you're allergic to erythromycin or it's not working, your dermatologist may prescribe another oral antibiotic that can be used in pregnancy.

Drugs that may be harmful to developing fetuses

The FDA classifies some topical and oral medications as pregnancy category C drugs. This categorization means that it's not known whether the medication will be harmful to an unborn baby. But, when it comes to benzoyl peroxide, sulfacetamide, and sulfur drugs, they've been around for ages and no evidence has ever shown them to be harmful to a fetus. With some of the other drugs mentioned below, definitive evidence isn't available one way or the other, so I recommend that you avoid them unless your healthcare provider or dermatologist says otherwise.

The following acne topicals have been used for many years and are probably safe to apply during pregnancy and nursing:

✔ **Benzoyl peroxide:** This drug has been around for generations. It's very effective for treating acne and can be purchased over the counter (see Chapters 7 and 9 where I talk about topical treatments and the numerous benzoyl peroxide products that are available). There have never been reports of problems that came from using benzoyl peroxide during pregnancy.

However, even though benzoyl peroxide is generally considered to be safe to use during pregnancy, you should be aware that the FDA classifies it in pregnancy category C. It's also not known whether benzoyl peroxide passes into breast milk. Because this product has been around for so long, when it was approved, the FDA didn't require that it be tested to the extent that drugs are nowadays.

If you're pregnant or breastfeeding your baby, you shouldn't use benzoyl peroxide topical without first talking to your doctor. You can then decide if the risks are low enough and the benefits are high enough for you to use it.

If during pregnancy or breastfeeding, you're advised to use a benzoyl peroxide combination product, it's probably wisest to use one that contains erythromycin such as Benzamycin Gel, rather than one that contains clindamycin, which I discuss later in this section.

✔ **Sulfacetamide/sulfur combinations:** As with benzoyl peroxide products, these pregnancy category C agents have been
used safely for many years. Combinations of sulfacetamide
and sulfur are contained in such products as Rosula, Rosac,
Rosanil, Nicosyn, and Novacet.

These medications should be used only when clearly needed
during pregnancy. Discuss the risks and benefits with your
doctor. These medications may pass into breast milk, so breastfeeding while using these medications isn't recommended.

The following FDA pregnancy category C topicals are "newer kids
on the block" and aren't recommended for use during pregnancy:

✔ **Topical retinoids:** These consist of tretinoin, Retin-A, Differin,
Tazorac, and Avita. Even though there is minimal absorption
of topical retinoids that can potentially reach a fetus, and
there's no evidence that these agents can harm an unborn
child, you should stop applying them once you think that
you're pregnant.

✔ **Clindamycin:** Prescription products that contain this antibiotic include Cleocin-T, as well as several generics. The effects
of clindamycin during pregnancy haven't been adequately
studied. Clindamycin combined with benzoyl peroxide is also
found in the combination products Benzaclin Gel and Duac
Gel (see Chapter 9).

Because clindamycin may appear in breast milk and could
affect a nursing infant, it's probably not advisable to use
products containing it if you are pregnant or plan to become
pregnant.

✔ **Aczone Gel:** This agent contains dapsone. There is minimal
absorption of this drug in the bloodstream when it's applied
topically; however, it's known that dapsone is excreted in
human milk when taken orally. I talk about this new drug in
Chapter 9.

Clindamycin and benzoyl peroxide are also found in the combination products Benzaclin Gel and Duac Gel (see Chapter 9).

Oral drugs known to cause birth defects

I recommend avoiding all oral medicines to treat acne when you're
pregnant. However, an oral penicillin derivative, such as amoxicillin (if you're not allergic to it), may be taken safely if your acne is
really bad. If you're allergic to penicillin or it's not working, your
dermatologist may prescribe another oral antibiotic that can be
used in pregnancy.

Many oral drugs can harm your unborn baby. In these cases, clear evidence exists that your child may have serious birth defects if you use them. The following medications must be avoided if you're pregnant or if you're contemplating becoming pregnant:

- **Tetracycline:** Tetracycline and its derivatives, minocycline and doxycycline, may cause some inhibition of bone growth and discoloration of teeth in a fetus. Tetracycline and its side effects are covered in Chapter 10.

- **Hormones:** The anti-androgens such as spironolactone that are sometimes used to treat acne, can, by blocking testosterone, interfere with the normal development of a male fetus and cause feminization. (See Chapter 11.)

- **Oral isotretinoin (Accutane):** Oral isotretinoin (eye-so-tret-ih-*no*-in) available as Accutane, Roaccutane, Amnesteem, Claravis, and Sotret, is a powerful drug that's used to treat severe nodular acne in carefully selected patients. This drug can cause severe fetal abnormalities. I discuss Accutane and its generics in Chapter 13.

There are many restrictions currently in place regarding oral isotretinoin, and with understandable cause. Oral isotretinoin can cause serious birth defects to infants born to women exposed to them. They should never — not under any circumstances — be taken during pregnancy! Even if a woman becomes pregnant within one month after stopping the drug, problems can still occur.

There also is an increased risk of miscarriage, premature births, and infant death associated with taking oral isotretinoin during pregnancy.

A recently published Swedish study showed an increased occurrence of certain heart defects in children born to mothers who had taken *oral* erythromycin in early pregnancy (first trimester). But it can't be certain that factors other than erythromycin didn't contribute to the increase in malformations. In the same study, the risk after treatment with penicillin demonstrated no increase in these malformations.

You're never too young

When acne appears in newborns it is known as *acne neonatorum*. It's actually very common. This type of acne is seen mainly in male infants and is believed to occur from the stimulation of an infant's sebaceous glands by maternal androgens. Most often, it requires no treatment because it usually goes away by itself.

The lesions of acne neonatorum usually appear at about 2 weeks of age. They consist of tiny red bumps and pustules that are seen on the cheeks, forehead, chin, neck, and sometimes the chest. They tend to appear over the course of a few weeks and often vanish over the course of a few months as the baby's large sebaceous glands become smaller and less active.

Treatment, if necessary, has traditionally been with benzoyl peroxide; however, recent studies have shown that a topical antifungal cream known as ketoconazole has been shown to be effective. It can be purchased over the counter as Nizoral cream.

Infantile acne can show up in children between the ages of 3 to 6 months of age. It's different than acne neonatorum because it more closely resembles teenage acne — the acne may appear as inflammatory as well as comedonal lesions.

In some instances, infantile acne has led to pitted scarring, and there's some evidence that this type of acne may be an indication of future problems with acne during adolescence. Treatment of infantile acne usually consists of topical benzoyl peroxide or a topical retinoid. Rarely, oral isotretinoin may be given for very severe potentially scarring cases.

If treatment of acne neonatorum or infantile acne is required, consult your pediatrician, and if necessary, ask to see a dermatologist. I tell you how to go about seeing a dermatologist in Chapter 8.

You're never too old

Some women pass through menopause without outgrowing their acne. Yes — acne during and after menopause! Just when you felt certain that the years of pimples have faded from your skin and your memory, they're back! No, you're not going through a second adolescence, it's those pesky hormones again! Although hormonally influenced acne typically begins around age 20 to 25, acne can persist in women over the age of 40 and continue into the peri-menopausal and menopausal periods.

Along with all the other changes that you go through during this time, acne just seems to add insult to injury. Post-menopausal acne isn't a common occurrence, but when estrogen levels begin to taper off and testosterone becomes the dominant hormone, acne — usually mild — can appear.

Facing Acne As an Adult Man

The good news for most adult men is that acne that *first* appears after age 20 is an unusual occurrence. I suppose the bad news is that if you're reading this, you're having just such an "unusual occurrence." In men with adult acne, lesions are more often seen on the chest and back. When it arises on the back, it's sometimes playfully called "backne." If you're a guy, and you're facing acne, odds are that one of several things is occurring:

✔ **The teen version has stuck around:** Though most acne vulgaris (teenage acne) clears up by the time you approach the 20 mark, it can stick around. Check out Chapter 4 for an explanation of acne vulgaris.

✔ **You're an athlete:** In recent years, acne is being seen increasingly on the chests and backs of men who participate in vigorous athletic activities. Some observers speculate that sweating and friction causes the acne because the primary sites are most often under clothing.

✔ **You've used performance-enhancing drugs:** Another, more likely, source of chest and back acne may result from the use of performance-enhancing preparations that contain such ingredients such as creatine, colostrum, and, of course, anabolic steroids such as testosterone and andro. I talk more about steroids in Chapter 6.

✔ **You don't really have acne:** If you have any doubt about your diagnosis, see a dermatologist because she may tell you that you don't have acne at all but may have rosacea, an adult acne look-alike, or *folliculitis* (an inflammation of hair follicles) due to shaving your face and maybe even from shaving your chest and back. (See Chapters 18 and 19 to learn more about these acne impostors.)

Significant scarring from acne is more common in men than in women. In men, lesions that leave scars may be the dominant type present, especially in men who had severe acne in their teens. In Chapter 16, I explain the types of scars and tell you what can be done about them.

Chapter 6

Evaluating Other Causes and Contributors: Myth and Reality

● ●

In This Chapter

▶ Exploring dirt and oil

▶ Revisiting your diet: Is your face what you eat?

▶ Looking at the connection between stress and acne

▶ Aggravating your acne

▶ Makeup: Does your face become what you put on it?

● ●

*A*s long as people have had acne, they've tried to find something to blame for the condition — including dirt, diet, stress, makeup, and sex. Although dermatologists and researchers still aren't 100 percent sure about what causes acne, we've come a long way in recent decades, and most doctors agree that hormones and heredity are the fundamental sources that lead to the development of acne (as I explain in Chapters 3 through 5).

In this chapter, I explore the role that stress and diet play in causing acne or making existing acne worse. I also review some of the medications and "tripwires" that have been implicated as causing or worsening acne. I end with an appraisal of the relationship between makeup and acne.

This chapter also looks at some of the historical misconceptions that have persisted about acne. For example, you've probably been warned not to eat too much chocolate. And you may have heard "The Big Bang Theory," that is, keep your hair away from your skin. Not true.

These types of myths are passed down from one family member to another, told to you by a friend, and occasionally published in beauty magazines. Myths die hard and often there is some underlying truth that can be found to explain where and how some of them got started; other times they're just based on silly folklore.

Debunking Dirt and Grease Theories

The appearance of acne — the black color of blackheads and facial oiliness — suggests that if only you rubbed and scrubbed your face really hard and often, you could get your acne to go away. Not so — in fact, before all of the effective acne treatments became available to us, that was how acne was often treated — and unsuccessfully I might add.

 What may look like dirt inside your blackheads is actually melanin, the pigment that provides the natural color of your skin. Despite what you may have seen or heard in commercials, your pores don't get blocked from the top down; instead, most of the action of acne formation takes place on the inside of your skin in your hair follicle (see Chapter 3 where I tell you the whole story).

Think about it. If dirt was a major reason that some people get acne, we'd probably see gazillions of blackheads, whiteheads, and pimples on the faces of folks who do a lot of manual labor such as coal miners, ditch diggers, construction workers, and gardeners. But it so happens that office workers, teachers, and doctors — even alas, dermatologists and their kids — get acne.

As for the oil, although there is a connection between how severe acne is and the amount of oil a person's skin produces, not all people with oily skin have acne and not all people with acne have oily skin. It so happens that some people with dry skin also have it.

Scrubbing and rubbing a face that has acne will only serve to irritate and redden an already inflamed complexion. Instead, the face should be washed daily (twice a day at the most!) with a gentle cleanser. For detailed information on proper face washing technique, see Chapter 2.

Dismissing the Diet — For the Most Part

We aren't *always* what we eat. Despite occasional personal anecdotes and persistent cultural myths, acne is probably not significantly influenced by diet.

In fact, there have been studies in which people were *actually paid* to eat chocolate. Yum! The conclusion: The chocolate-eating subjects' acne didn't get worse. Furthermore, several substances found in chocolate have been identified as being mood-lifters that apparently increase your brain's *endorphins* (chemicals that decrease pain and elevate your mood). So chocolate isn't bad for your blemishes; your stress level may diminish and so may your pimples! However, your waistline may get wider.

Currently, there is some disagreement about the link between diet and acne; several researchers are suggesting that there may be a degree of truth behind some dietary factors having an influence on acne. For example, certain dairy products and refined sugars that are found in our Western diet are now being evaluated as possible acne triggers. The jury is still out on this issue.

In the meantime, if you're absolutely convinced that a certain food type is making your acne worse — avoid it! But if your acne is being treated properly, you probably don't need to worry about food affecting it.

Take a skeptical approach with any acne "cure" books that hype a special diet, such as salmon, as one of the fundamental treatment components.

Frying up an acne fable

To prevent pimples, you may have been told to avoid junk food because it contains so much fat and grease that it'll make your skin greasy too and you'll get whopper-sized McPimples!

According to studies to date, it's the oil in your sebaceous glands that causes you problems and *not* the oil in your French fries or in your stomach. Sure, it makes sense to follow a healthy diet, which involves avoiding greasy foods, but avoiding such foods doesn't guarantee a clear complexion.

Here's the beef — and the milk

Many cattle are fed androgens to help them build muscle. And as you may have read in Chapter 3, your body's androgens are often what kick-starts the overproduction of oil. Some researchers are looking into whether we also get androgenic stimulation and acne when we eat beef. On the other hand, the androgens may be degraded by cooking before they get to our acne-prone, androgen-sensitive hair follicles.

And there are some investigators (a small minority, mind you) who believe that milk, particularly skim milk, and some other dairy products may worsen — or even cause — acne. They claim that the androgenic hormones that are injected into our cows to make them produce more milk get into our bodies and give us pimples. But it's questionable whether the hormones in milk could survive the high levels of *gastric acidity* (our stomach acid) and be absorbed into our bodies.

My take on this debate is simple: I've seen many vegetarians who choose not to eat any flesh foods (fish, chicken, beef), and a few vegans (pronounced *vee*-guns), people that totally avoid eating any animal products including dairy and eggs. Guess what — both vegans and vegetarians still get acne like the rest of us! (And by the way, when was the last time you saw a cow with pimples?)

So right now, nobody knows for sure, but for the time being, I think you should listen to the age old parental advice and drink your milk! (Unless you have a milk allergy.) Same with eating that steak. The jury is out on the whole cow-androgen-acne thing.

No, it's the sweets: A disease of Western civilization?

A recent study regarding two societies, the Kitavan Islanders of Papua New Guinea and the Aché hunter gatherers of Paraguay, found absolutely no evidence of acne until these groups were exposed to a Western diet. The investigators of this article (found in the December 2002 volume of the *Archives of Dermatology*) suggested that the refined sugar in our Western diets is a possible cause of acne.

Bottom line: Besides diet, there are so many other factors that might be responsible for their lack of acne, such as climate, sun exposure, and less stress in their tropical homeland.

And even when American diets were much lower in sweets 30 years ago, teens probably had as much acne as today.

No, it's the iodides

It has been traditionally believed that overeating foods that are rich in iodides, such as sushi, seaweed, and shellfish, can cause or aggravate acne. Bottom line: As far as I know, there have been no reports of acne epidemics reported so far in Japan or Korea.

Salmon saves the day, or does it?

There are those who advocate eating more fish, most notably, salmon, which is loaded with the anti-inflammatory omega-3 fatty acid. Its fans would have you believe that eating salmon can help you prevent and treat acne.

Decoupling the acne-sex links

A patient of mine made the following comments, "Recently, I woke up to find my face covered with acne. I'm 18 years old and I get a zit now and then, but I can't ever remember having a breakout this bad (at least 20 pimples) appearing overnight! I tried to recall anything that might have caused this, and my only guess is that I also have been having sex lately. Is there some weird kind of hormone thing that's doing this to me? I thought sex was supposed to cure your pimples!"

This gentleman was misguided on a number of accounts. Not so long ago, it was believed that the absence of sexual activity caused acne. Having "normal" sexual relations during marriage was held to be a "natural treatment" for acne. Though this form of therapy may sound appealing, there is no evidence that it works. This idea probably stems from the fact people traditionally got married in their early 20s, about the same time that acne usually burns itself out.

And although the androgenic "sex" hormones are a primary cause of acne, you don't necessarily develop acne because you have too much of this hormone or from sex. Likewise, some folks still think that masturbation causes acne. This idea, originating as early as the 17th century to dissuade young people from having premarital sex, is just plain silly. The only connection between masturbation and acne is that both are associated with adolescence. Moralists blamed many diseases, including blindness, deafness, and terrible skin eruptions, on such "wicked" practices. Don't believe it! The guilt that surrounds masturbation in the minds of many teenagers is probably responsible for this timeworn myth.

Eating more salmon is likely a good idea for your general health. However, farmed salmon may contain PCBs and dioxins, two substances that have been linked to various health problems. And wild salmon contains mercury. So don't eat too much of it.

Understanding Stress and Acne

Modern-day living, anxiety in the workplace, too many or too few hormones, nuclear threats, terrorism, inflation, crime, poverty, obesity — it's enough to give you terminal acne!

 Most investigators agree that stress *doesn't cause* acne; however, most would agree that stress *seems* to worsen it. Just ask college students at exam time, teenagers about to go to the prom, or someone going for that first job interview.

It's well known that at times of stress, the body releases excess amounts of *glucocorticoids* (the body's natural steroids). Some people think that the glucocorticoids, having some androgenic properties (see the next section where I talk about glucocorticoids when they're taken orally), cause sebaceous glands to secrete more oil and thus worsen acne or even cause an acnelike eruption.

It has been suggested that regular stress-reducing activity (like exercise, knitting, yoga, and so forth) can help minimize the glucocorticoids, and reduce their effect on sebaceous glands.

Some pundits also advise getting extra sleep and meditating. Just like with diet and acne, there is no hard evidence that these measures really do much to help reduce acne. However, they *are* healthy habits that may reduce stress, so why not? See Chapter 15 where I cover some of these approaches.

Addressing some Aggravating Agents

A host of outside agents such as drugs, physical factors such as cosmetics, and even sun exposure have been considered to be triggers and tripwires for acne. I review these agents in the next section. In particular, certain drugs can be *acnegenic* (acne producing) or create skin eruptions that look exactly like acne *(acneiform reactions)*. The same drugs can sometimes exacerbate pre-existing acne.

Drugs that can induce acne

Acne reactions caused by medications are usually *self-limiting,* which means they disappear when the drugs are stopped. If the drug must be taken for an extended period of time, the acne or acnelike lesions can be treated with the same medications that are used to fight most forms of acne.

Corticosteroids

Oral corticosteroids are synthetic derivatives of the natural steroid, cortisol, which is produced by the adrenal glands. They're prescribed for a large number of serious inflammatory diseases. They're called "systemic" steroids if taken by mouth or given by injection as opposed to topical corticosteroids (see the next section), which are applied directly to the skin. Prednisone, prednisolone, and methylprednisolone are examples.

These drugs sometimes produce inflammatory acne lesions consisting of papules or pustules that have a tendency to appear on the chest and/or back (sometimes called *steroid folliculitis*). They disappear after the medication is stopped. Comedones (blackheads and whiteheads) are generally absent from steroid-induced acne.

The overuse of potent *topical corticosteroids* (used for many skin conditions) on the face can cause a condition similar to acne. It is known as *steroid-induced rosacea.* I discuss this condition and its treatment in Chapter 18.

I realize that this sounds somewhat contradictory, since the oral corticosteroid drugs are *anti-inflammatory,* and it would appear that they would actually be used to *treat* acne. If fact, they are used for acne treatment under special circumstances. Sometimes they're used to treat the nodules and scars of acne by injection. I describe these situations in Chapter 16. And on special occasions, we dermatologists prescribe corticosteroids orally for short three-to-five-day, low-dose "bursts" as an "emergency" treatment to wipe out acne for a special occasion (wedding, prom, and so on). They can really wipe out acne fast, but only for short periods of time.

Anabolic-androgenic steroids

Abuse of these hormones can lead to acne and other serious health problems. Besides legitimate medical uses of androgens such as testosterone for hormone deficiencies, widespread use and abuse of these compounds exist, particularly the *anabolic-androgenic steroids,* as performance-enhancing drugs.

This type of acne is observed in males mainly on their backs, shoulders, and chest, and less often on the face, whereas in female athletes using these drugs, lesions tend to appear on the face as well as on the back and shoulders. An already-existing acne problem may get worse or nonexisting acne may be evoked.

Androstenedione

Androstenedione (andro) is a hormone produced by the adrenal glands, ovaries, and testes. It's a precursor hormone that's normally converted in the body to testosterone and estrogen in both men and women. Andro made the news after the former baseball player Mark McGwire admitted taking it around the time of his record-breaking home run season. Although ads claim that andro-containing supplements promote increased muscle mass, studies have shown that andro poses the same kinds of health hazards as anabolic steroids. The U.S Food and Drug Administration (FDA) cautions about the risks for young people who take andro: acne, an early start of puberty, and stunted growth.

DHEA (dehydroepiandrosterone)

This hormone, sometimes billed as the "fountain of youth" hormone, is also a steroid hormone, a chemical cousin of testosterone and estrogen. Because DHEA is converted into testosterone, it has been noted to produce excessive facial and body hair, besides causing acne.

Other oral medications

Other drugs that have been observed to have acnegenic properties include:

- Lithium
- Iodine
- Isoniazid
- Diphenylhydantoin
- Certain androgenic contraceptive pills (see Chapter 11)

Initiating or irritating factors?

In this section, I list some of the activities, exposures, or things done to the skin that have historically been reported to bring on or exacerbate acne.

Acne cosmetica

This condition is described as a persistent, low-grade type of acne usually involving the chin and cheeks of women who use cosmetics. The lesions arise primarily as closed comedones as well as papules and pustules. It is often thought to be caused by *comedogenic* (blackhead- and whitehead-producing) substances in the cosmetics. In all likelihood, however, these folks probably have adult-onset acne, and they just happen to use the cosmetics to hide the acne lesions — and of course, the cosmetics get the blame for causing the acne!

Because most major cosmetics are noncomedogenic — meaning they don't cause acne — this type of acne is unlikely to be seen much, if at all, nowadays.

Pomade acne

A variant of cosmetic acne, known as pomade acne, can occur if greases, like oils, Vaseline, cocoa butter, and hair oils are used to style hair or are applied to the skin. If pomade or hair oil spreads onto the forehead, it can block pores, causing comedones.

Pomade acne is almost exclusively seen in African-Americans and usually appears on the forehead and temples. I discuss this type of acne in Chapter 12. Treatment consists of avoiding pomades. If you must continue using a pomade, try applying it to the ends of the hair only to avoid contact with the scalp and hairline. See the color section of this book for a visual.

Sunlight and acne (Mallorca acne)

Also called *acne estivalis* ("estivalis" means summer); this is a rare form of acne that occurs in the summer or following a vacation in the sun. This condition is so rare that I don't think I've seen a case of it.

But I have seen the damaging results that excessive exposure to the sun can have on both healthy skin and skin with teenage and adult-onset acne. For more on this issue, see Chapter 14, which also discusses potentially beneficial types of light therapy for acne, and Chapter 22.

Acne mechanica

This variation of acne is due to mechanical factors, including friction, sweating, and pressure. It is provoked by such factors as chin straps, bra straps, articles of clothing, orthopedic casts, backpacks, chairs, and car or bus seats. The acne is seen at the sites where these items rub and persistently press against the skin, such as under a chin strap or cast. This type of acne is often simply an aggravation of the existing lesions of acne or an inflammation of hair follicles known as *folliculitis*.

Acne detergens

This refers to the aggravation of the existing lesions of acne by too frequent washing with comedogenic soaps and rough cloths and abrasive pads. It certainly can be irritating, but overwashing doesn't cause acne.

Dioxins and Agent Orange (chloracne)

Agent Orange, an herbicide, was used during the war in Vietnam. Some veterans reported a variety of health problems and concerns attributed to exposure to this agent, including chloracne.

Agent Orange contains *dioxins* (halogenated aromatic hydrocarbons), a group of chemicals known to increase the likelihood of cancer. The first disease associated with dioxins was the extreme skin disease chloracne. It causes acnelike pustules on the body that can and do last for several years and result in significant scarring.

It develops a few months after swallowing, inhaling, or touching the responsible agent.

Most cases are due to occupational exposure, but it can also arise after accidental environmental poisoning. Deliberate dioxin poisoning is blamed for Ukrainian President Victor Yushchenko's dramatically changed appearance during the "Orange Revolution" in 2004.

Making Up and Breaking Out?

Makeup doesn't *cause* acne. *Acne cosmetica* (see the related section earlier in the chapter) is the traditional name for the type of acne that cosmetics supposedly cause. I realize that some reactions to cosmetics can sometimes look like inflammatory acne, but it's really just your skin reacting negatively to one or more of the ingredients found in your makeup that makes already-existing acne get redder and look worse.

And between you and me — I don't believe that cosmetics have much to do in the development or worsening of acne!! There, I've said it.

I generally tell my patients, "If you're happy with your cosmetics, stay with them; if you feel that your cosmetics are causing or worsening your acne, just stop using them for a few weeks and see if the bumps go away!"

Testing, testing: What's up, Doc?

The ear of the rabbit is very sensitive. Besides bringing good luck (oh, that's the foot, isn't it?) and warding off danger, the rabbit's ear, for decades, has been used to test cosmetic ingredients to see whether they cause *comedones* (blackheads and whiteheads). Substances known to be *acnegenic* (acne-producing) in humans will rapidly produce comedones in rabbit ears.

However, the rabbit ear differs from human skin and may not be an accurate model of the human face, because humans and rabbits don't necessary respond in the same way to cosmetics application.

Because of these difficulties, more recent approaches used by cosmetic companies often test makeup on the upper backs of male volunteers who have acne. Again, it may be difficult to relate a man's back to a woman's face.

By the way, when was the last time you saw a rabbit wearing makeup?

However, there are plenty of folks who disagree with me, some of whom are fellow dermatologists. In the next sections, I tell you what others have to say. I present the information to be inclusive and present the traditional belief that makeup and cosmetics are very important issues when it comes to acne.

Reading the ingredients

Nowadays, most cosmetic products boast of being non-pore-clogging and "oil free." And most of them have a label that states that the product has been tested and verified as being noncomedogenic. It's on virtually every label on every cosmetic product.

However, some skin-care products are considered to be *comedogenic,* which means they cause whiteheads and blackheads. The damaging effect of cosmetics on acne has been attributed to the presence of excess oil in such cosmetics.

What ingredients in the leading cosmetic products are believed by some dermatologists to cause acne? The following three are considered to be the leading candidates:

- ✔ **Lanolin:** This is oil from the skin of sheep. It's similar to the fatty acids found in human skin.

- ✔ **Isopropyl myristate:** This substance adds "slip," which makes a product go on the skin smoother and causes a slick sheer feel. There are a number of chemicals similar to isopropyl myristate, including isopropyl isostearate, butyl stearate, octyl stearate, and laureth-4.

✔ **D & C red dyes:** These dyes derived from coal tars are also believed to be comedogenic.

Although some experts believe these ingredients are acne-causing, I don't personally believe they cause acne. However, if your acne seems to get worse when wearing cosmetics, look for these ingredients on the label of your current products. Try new products that don't contain them to see whether your skin condition improves.

Living in an oil-free world

Is your cosmetic really, absolutely oil free? On the assumption that sebum is a beneficial component of the skin, chemists have tried to imitate this substance, but the "oil free" claim isn't exactly valid and can be misleading because the oil substitutes that are used in these products are synthetic and are considered to be more harmful than the excess sebum found in the skin that can block pores.

The alleged bad guys

Generally speaking, the most acne-causing cosmetics are:

✔ Foundation makeup

✔ Pressed powders

✔ Thick creams

✔ Blushers

Moisturizers can also be a source of acne-producing substances. In order to make these moisturizing products smooth onto the skin easily, they're often manufactured with ingredients such as acetylated lanolin, searic acid, and cetyl alcohol. All of these ingredients are considered to be comedogenic.

The alleged good guys

The recommended moisturizers are those that have a base of petrolatum or mineral oil. Powder blushers are usually preferred over creams, and cream/powder foundations are usually preferred over the liquid type because loose powders help to "mop up" the oil. If a liquid foundation is chosen, it should be silicone-based (containing cyclomethicone or dimethicone).

Chapter 7

Taking Care of Acne Over the Counter

*A*n enormous multi-billion-dollar industry exists with the intention of treating your acne and competing for your money. Just look at all the items that pack the shelves of drugstores, supermarkets, and chain stores. They come in fancy, eye-catching packages, as soaps, cleansers, lotions, pads, creams, gels, ointments, wipes, foams, and masks, and offer a treasure trove of preparations: oil-free, hypoallergenic, organic, non-comedogenic, herbal, radiant, protein rich, dermatologist-tested, and so on. No wonder people who treat their acne themselves are so often and so easily overwhelmed and confused about what product is right for them. But I'm here to clear things up. (In more ways than one!)

In this chapter, I talk about ways that you can go it alone — especially if your acne is mild. In the process, I list and describe the *over-the-counter,* or *OTC, medications* (no prescription neces-sary) that may help you along the way, and I help you figure out which ones work and which ones don't. But self-treatment isn't the right solution for everyone. So if you haven't perused Chapter 1, you may want to do so to determine whether self-treatment is a good idea for you or whether you should just head straight to the doctor's office.

Mirror, mirror on the wall . . .

Nobody looks at your skin as closely as you do. And maybe you facilitate matters by using a magnifying mirror that helps you see every little spot and pore in your skin. Everything looks gigantic. Your face looks like the surface of the moon and each pore looks like the Grand Canyon!

But unless you're being scrutinized by a curious cosmetologist, evaluated for one of those real-life makeover shows on television, or you're married to Sherlock Holmes, nobody else is going to look at your skin with a magnifying lens! You're the victim of your own supercritical eye. Besides, other people are probably thinking about what they saw in *their* mirror this morning. So do something better with your time — go for a walk, ask for a raise, take up the violin, or go skydiving.

Taking Action Topically: A Primer

A *topical* product is one that is applied on the skin, such as a cream, ointment, gel, foam, or lotion. Almost every OTC acne medication is topical rather than *oral,* taken by mouth. Topical therapy is generally safer than *systemic* (oral or injected) therapy.

Topical acne treatments (both the OTC and prescription varieties) are made up of two general types of ingredients that you find on all labels:

- ✔ **Active ingredient:** This part of the medication does the real grunt work. I recommend you start your search for an OTC treatment by looking at the active ingredient because it's the most important component of a product. Most commonly found are benzoyl peroxide, salicylic acid, sulfur, and resorcinol. You can read more about these ingredients in the section "Getting In on the Active Ingredients."

- ✔ **Inactive ingredient(s):** This part of the medicine is the stuff that holds onto the medicine and preserves it, keeps the product moving easily through the container, and makes the medicine easier to apply. Inactive ingredients are sometimes referred to as the *inert ingredient* or the *vehicle* because they deliver the medicine. You can read more about these ingredients in the section "The Lazy Bums! Inactive Ingredients."

In choosing the right topical treatment, you need to consider both active and inactive ingredients. Just as some active ingredients may be more beneficial for your particular acne, certain vehicles may be more conducive to your skin type. The rest of this chapter explains what the various active ingredients do and how you use them. I also explain what type of delivery vehicle is best for your particular skin type.

Don't buy brand-name products when you can spend less on generic. That way, you don't have to pay for the fancy packaging and marketing that the name brands put into their products!

After you start to treat your acne, don't get into the routine of checking your face every day and looking for improvement. The treatments take time to start working — sometimes up to six to eight weeks, so be patient!

The Lazy Bums! Inactive Ingredients

Skin looks and feels better when it's not too oily or too dry. If your skin tends to be dry, a moisturizing base (vehicle) is best; if it's very oily, select a product that has a drying base. Of course, if you have neither dry nor oily skin, choose a neutral product that's neither moisturizing nor drying. Most topical treatments fall into one of a few different categories, based on their delivery vehicles. Table 7-1 lists the most commonly used vehicles for delivering effective topical acne treatments. Look for your skin type there.

The inactive ingredients don't do anything to fight acne, but some may be better for you than others based on your skin type. One delivery agent doesn't fit all. If you have oily skin or if you have dry or sensitive skin, you may have to experiment with different preparations.

Table 7-1	Matching Bases and Faces	
Vehicle (Base)	*Best for This Skin*	*Description*
Alcohol solutions	Oily	Evaporate quickly. The most drying of all these treatments and can be very irritating. Cover large areas easily.
Aqueous solutions	Normal to dry	These are water based and alcohol-free. They're less drying and irritating than alcohol solutions. Cover large areas easily.

(continued)

Table 7-1 *(continued)*

Vehicle (Base)	Best for This Skin	Description
Creams	Normal to oily	Generally more popular than ointments because they're less greasy. Often preferred by patients because they absorb into the skin quickly. Their water content makes them more drying than ointments.
Foams	Normal to oily	May be somewhat drying, but they're easy to spread, particularly on hairy areas such as chests and backs of males. Very expensive.
Gels	Normal to oily	Essentially oil-free and have a mildly drying effect. Some of the newer gel preparations contain emollients such as glycerin and dimethicone, which help diminish the drying effects.
Lotions	Any	May be somewhat moisturizing; however, those that contain propylene glycol may have drying effects. Easy to apply.
Ointment	Normal to dry	Greasy. More lubricating and tend to be less irritating than creams and gels.

If you have combination skin that has an oily T-zone and a dry lower face, you might have to use different vehicles for different parts of your face.

As for cleansers, washes, and scrubs, I think they're somewhat overrated, because most of them hardly have enough time to do anything. They get rinsed off before they can really penetrate and do the job!

How much cream, ointment, or lotion should you apply? For those of us old enough to remember the old hair cream commercial: A little dab will do you. Think thin, not thick; a little works as well as a lot. Don't be inclined to have a "more is better" tendency. Only the thin layer that is actually in contact with the skin gets absorbed; the remainder is either rubbed off or unnecessary.

Gobbing it on is wasteful, and besides, it takes longer to rub it in and make it vanish!

Getting In on the Active Ingredients

If you spend a little time comparing the labels on the products you find at the drugstore, you discover how incredibly similar they all are — just about all of them contain one of the following active ingredients plus other inactive ingredients:

✔ Benzoyl peroxide

✔ Salicylic acid

✔ Sulfur

✔ Resorcinol

Finding topical products that work is easier than you may suppose. The active ingredient you choose depends on what kind of acne you have:

✔ If your acne consists mostly of blackheads and whiteheads, get a product that contains benzoyl peroxide and then, if necessary, add one that has salicylic acid in it.

✔ If you're just starting to get a few zits (inflammatory papules), try benzoyl peroxide alone.

In the following sections, I tell you about benzoyl peroxide and salicylic acid, as well other *less active* active ingredients that don't work so well.

The benefits of benzoyl peroxide

Benzoyl peroxide, a potent antibacterial agent that kills *P. acnes,* the bacteria that are involved in producing acne, is the most commonly used OTC acne medication, and for good reason — it works!

Benzoyl peroxide dries and peels the skin and removes dead cells, helps to clear blocked follicles, the non-inflammatory comedones (blackheads and whiteheads), and it works on the papules and pustules. A triple threat!

Unlike antibiotics and other prescription medications, you can use benzoyl peroxide for months, even years at a time, and there are really no long-term side effects including *tolerance* (bacterial resistance) associated with it. (For more on tolerance, see Chapter 10.)

You can find benzoyl peroxide in many brand-name OTC products, such as Clearasil, Oxy, Clean and Clear, PanOxyl, and Neutrogena, as well as less-expensive generic or store brand products. You can also find it in creams, gels, lotions, foams, soaps, washes, masks, and scrubs and in combination with other topical products.

Here are a couple of little tidbits to keep in mind:

✔ Of all the benzoyl-peroxide options, creams, lotions, and pads are more effective than washes, soaps, and scrubs.

✔ Benzoyl peroxide is available as a prescription (see Chapter 9), but prescription benzoyl peroxide formulations are no more effective than OTC products, they just cost more.

Using benzoyl peroxide

Benzoyl peroxide is designed to treat existing acne and prevent future breakouts. If you have acne vulgaris, you should use it even when your face is clear. Women can use it regularly to prevent or minimize hormone-related acne breakouts.

The strength of benzoyl peroxide varies in the different products, ranging from 2.5 to 10.0 percent. Lower strength benzoyl peroxide preparations, such as 2.5 percent, are less irritating than the higher strength 5 percent and 10 percent concentrations and are just as effective for most people, plus they're cheaper! Start out using the lowest dose possible, and then move up in strength if you need to. You minimize the chances of irritation and hopefully save some money.

In general, you begin using benzoyl peroxide products sparingly and then work toward more frequent application (follow the instructions that accompany the package — if you don't understand them, ask your pharmacist, nurse, or doctor to explain them to you). Here are some general guidelines:

1. **Start out doing this every other night. After you wash your face, sparingly apply a very thin layer to areas of your skin that have acne or are acne-prone.**

   Avoid your eyes, lips, and the corners of your mouth, which are often very sensitive.

2. **As you are able to tolerate it, build up to once or even twice daily if you're not making too much progress.**

When you choose a benzoyl peroxide treatment, keep these points in mind:

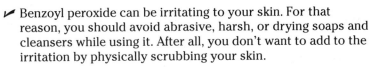

✔ Benzoyl peroxide can be irritating to your skin. For that reason, you should avoid abrasive, harsh, or drying soaps and cleansers while using it. After all, you don't want to add to the irritation by physically scrubbing your skin.

✔ Benzoyl peroxide can bleach hair, sheets, towels, and clothing. (It contains peroxide, a powerful bleach.) To avoid the bleaching effect, an old T-shirt should be worn after applying benzoyl peroxide to acne on the back or chest. Also, make sure the benzoyl peroxide has completely dried before the treated skin touches towels, clothes, or bedding (towels, sheets, and pillowcases should be white).

✔ You can apply makeup or other skin-care products, such as moisturizer, over benzoyl peroxide.

✔ Be patient, acne responds *very slowly* to treatment. It may take several months before you notice significant improvement. To prevent new lesions from forming, continue using benzoyl peroxide even after your acne clears.

Side effects

Dryness of the treated area can be expected and is usually mild. If your skin is visibly scaly, apply a light, non-oily moisturizer, like Eucerin Daily Control & Care Moisturizer, Cetaphil Moisturizing Lotion, or Olay Oil-Free Active Hydrating Beauty Fluid.

You may experience a mild burning sensation or reddening of the skin when you first start to apply benzoyl peroxide. Irritation and burning are common, but usually disappear in two to three weeks.

If the preparation you're applying causes too much redness, peeling, or dryness of your skin, reduce the number of times a day that you use it, or use a weaker strength. If necessary, discontinue using it altogether.

Use of benzoyl peroxide products may also cause *contact dermatitis* (red, dry, inflamed, itchy skin) due to irritation or allergy. It can be treated with a topical steroid such as a 1 percent hydrocortisone cream, which is available without a prescription. Look for the brand names Cortaid or Cortizone 10, or store brand equivalents.

Trying salicylic acid

By itself, in the low concentrations that are available over the counter, salicylic acid isn't very effective in treating acne. However, it's believed to help the skin absorb benzoyl peroxide and other more effective prescription topical acne medications.

Salicylic acid is a *beta-hydroxy acid (BHA)*. Beta-hydroxy acids are commonly called "fruit acids" because they're natural substances derived from fruits, sugar, and plants. They're found in many over-the-counter products.

Salicylic acid works by *exfoliating,* which means it removes the top layers of dead skin cells. Salicylic acid loosens the gluelike substances that hold the surface skin cells to each other, allowing the dead skin to peel off. It's also oil soluble and can get into oil-clogged pores. These actions help the skin renew itself faster and reduce the chance for pore blockage and a subsequent acne breakout.

The OTC products that contain only salicylic acid are, at best, minimally effective in treating non-inflammatory acne lesions (like blackheads and whiteheads). Salicylic acid doesn't have any effect on sebum production; it just removes the sebum that has reached the surface of the skin and makes your skin feel smoother. That's why salicylic acid is also found in some makeup removal products.

Much more powerful salicylic acid preparations are sometimes used by dermatologists and plastic surgeons as acne treatments and for wrinkle removing and skin rejuvenation procedures. The high concentrations are much more effective at clearing up blackheads and whiteheads than the OTC products (see Chapter 14).

As with benzoyl peroxide, salicylic acid comes in a host of formulations and is an ingredient in Clearasil, Oxy, Clean and Clear, PanOxyl, and Neutrogena, as well as less expensive generic brands.

Salicylic acid is available in concentrations from 0.5 to 2.0 percent, mainly in creams, lotions, pads, washes, cleansers, and astringents (agents that dry oily skin). It's available as a single agent or sometimes in combination with sulfur. (For more on using sulfur, see the section "Resorcinol and sulfur," later in this chapter.)

Creams, lotions, and pads that contain salicylic acid are more effective than the other options.

As part of their skin-care lines, the same companies that offer benzoyl peroxide products often offer products containing salicylic acid. Sometimes they're packaged together as a "total acne treatment system." When these "systems" contain salicylic acid as well as benzoyl peroxide as their active ingredients, they can work quite effectively to treat your acne.

Those expensive mail-order OTC combination "systems" that you see on TV infomercials can't always be trusted or tailored to match your skin. But if you really want to use one, you can buy a much, much cheaper "knockoff" variety at your local drugstore or Wal-Mart. Read the labels!

Using salicylic acid products

Salicylic acid products *are* appropriate starter treatments for children who are just beginning to develop mild comedonal acne. When used alone for other types of acne or more advanced acne, don't expect very much from them.

As with benzoyl peroxide, you apply a thin layer of salicylic acid to areas of skin affected by acne. If you discover that the salicylic acid isn't working very well, substitute or add a benzoyl peroxide product to your regimen.

Side effects

Dryness of the treated area can be expected and is usually mild. If these products are used with benzoyl peroxide formulations, the dryness and irritation can be more severe, and if the skin is visibly scaly, apply a light non-oily moisturizer such as one described in the section "Using benzoyl peroxide."

Other OTC medications

In this section, I briefly describe the medications that are of questionable value in treating your acne. Some can be quite expensive.

Retinols and alpha hydroxy acids

Retinol is a derivative of Vitamin A. You may have heard or read the term in advertising for products that claim to reduce fine lines and wrinkles by increasing cell turnover (sometimes called *rejuvenation*).

Retinols are sometimes used alone, or in combination with *alpha hydroxy acids* (AHAs). Glycolic acid is the AHA most frequently used for facial treatments, but lactic and citric acid are also used. (Most often AHAs are derived from fruits, which is why they're sometimes called "fruit acids." As you may expect, lactic acid doesn't come from fruit, it comes from milk.)

OTC products contain very low concentrations of AHA, which acts as a mild exfoliant. Although retinols and AHAs were originally marketed to fight aging skin, they're both currently being touted for use in treating acne; however, their effectiveness as an acne treatment hasn't been scientifically tested.

Chemical peels have become popular as anti-aging, facial rejuvenation procedures; however, they're sometimes used to treat acne and acne scars. This method involves the application of strong acid solutions such as AHAs or BHAs *(beta-hydroxy acids)*, which cause the skin to peel off and encourage regeneration of new skin. The treatment that is right for you depends on your skin type, and the activity of your acne. Such AHAs and BHAs that are applied and dispensed by physicians are much stronger than those that you can purchase over the counter. I discuss chemical peels in Chapter 14. The over-the-counter products have been proven to be effective for the treatment of acne.

Resorcinol and sulfur

The following agents have been used to treat acne for many generations without great success, but they're still available. Because they've been around for so long, I include them primarily for their historical interest and to tell you to save your money if you see these guys listed on a label:

- ✔ **Resorcinol:** This still-popular ingredient is frequently combined with sulfur in OTC products. Redness and peeling of your skin may occur after a few days.

- ✔ **Sulfur:** Sulfur has been used for more than 50 years in combination with other agents, such as alcohol, salicylic acid, and resorcinol. It is found in many OTC acne medications. Sulfur reacts with the skin in such a way that it makes it dry out, look red, and peel. Due to its unpleasant, "rotten egg" odor, sulfur isn't frequently used alone as an acne treatment.

Multi-ingredient products

You can find numerous products that include various combinations of benzoyl peroxide, resorcinol, aloe, glycolic acid, sulfur, and salicylic acid. Also, herbal remedies are available that contain aloe, lemon oil, and various other fruit-derived items. Such products are difficult to evaluate scientifically.

You're better off avoiding these products that contain such a hodgepodge of ingredients; besides, you only pay more for them.

Avoid OTC products that fall under the heading "herbal," "organic," or "natural." Their effectiveness has rarely been tested in clinical or scientific trials. The value of such treatments is generally unknown. In Chapter 15, I explore some of these "new age" treatments. And don't bother experimenting with some old home remedies such as rubbing on papaya or a paste of roasted pomegranate skin, fresh cut cloves of garlic, and so on. Fruits and vegetables don't work. They taste good, but are better put to work in your stomach than on your face. On second thought, I'm not so sure about the taste of pomegranate skin.

A Word about Acne Soaps, Cleansing Strips, Et Al

Some products physically (rather than chemically) agitate your skin. In most cases, they remove dirt, sebum, and dead skin cells from the surface, but they don't do much, if anything, to treat your acne. Having a clean face is great, but these rubby, scrubby products often only serve to irritate and redden an already inflamed complexion. Here are some of the most common physical acne treatments:

- **Pore cleansing strips:** These sticky patches temporarily lift solidified sebum and dead cells out of your pores for a day or so. They may occasionally cause mild irritation. They aren't very useful.

- **Acne soaps:** Antibacterial foaming washes, scrubs, and soap bars are available in many shapes and sizes. Some contain benzoyl peroxide, others have salicylic acid and some have triclosan, an antibacterial chemical cleanser that removes excess sebaceous secretions.

  None of them hang around on your skin long enough to do much to help your acne. To make them more effective, leave them on for at least 5 to 10 minutes before rinsing them off.

- **Exfoliants:** These are products that physically scrub the skin cells off. They can be very harsh on your skin if you have inflammatory acne, and they can be especially irritating when they contain salicylic acid. Exfoliants come in many forms: abrasive sponges, cosmetic scrubs, facial masks, toners, pads, and sponges. Avoid these products if you have sensitive skin.

- **Masks:** Masks to treat acne are essentially self-indulgent ways to spend more money and get a mild facial exfoliation. Masks contain various ingredients such as salicylic acid, benzoyl peroxide, vitamins, aloe, and lemon juice, to name a few.

- **Loofah sponges:** Almost as bad as using sandpaper on your skin if you have inflammatory acne. If you have non-inflammatory acne and tough skin, I guess they can't hurt.

These treatments are most effective when used sparingly and in conjunction with other treatments that have antibacterial properties, like benzoyl peroxide. But my final word on all of these products: Save your money! Go with proven treatments like benzoyl peroxide and salicylic acid preparations, if you're going to treat acne on your own.

Evaluating Advertisers' Claims

There is some excellent, time-tested, helpful information about acne and acne-fighting products available, but sadly you need to take a lot of the stuff you find with a grain of salt. Be especially wary of the following as you walk through acne aisle at the drugstore, search the Internet, visit your local bookstore, or watch those infomercials:

- ✔ **People who are selling products:** Many supposed experts have a financial interest in pushing their own products; this often outweighs their interest in really educating and helping you. So learn to read between the lines and to skip all of the hucksterism. Such keywords and phrases as *magic, revolutionary, our laboratories,* and *overnight* should have you raising a skeptical eyebrow.

- ✔ **Claims that are too good to be true:** Any product or book that has the word *cure* on the package or in its title, or *24 hours* or even *5 weeks to clear skin,* should make you very suspicious. I don't know how to cure acne and I'm a dermatologist with many powerful drugs at my disposal. There is no cure for acne, and in most instances, and even with the strongest of medications, it often takes months to get it under control and years of treatment to keep your skin clear.

- ✔ **Unsubstantiated claims about scientific testing:** When a product says it was *dermatologist-tested,* it wasn't necessarily approved or recommended by dermatologists. It could be that just *one* dermatologist tested it; maybe the dermatologist tested it and *didn't like it!* But I guess the manufacturer can still say that it was dermatologist tested. And when a highly paid TV actor/doctor or your favorite movie star or pop star endorses a product, I realize that it's not easy to separate the real claims from the phony. Perky ears, raised eyebrows, and this book (not very modest of me!) can be your best guides.

I've written this book to provide you with the information you need to make educated decisions about your acne. If you elect to go it alone in your acne treatment, your pharmacist is an excellent source of additional information to help you find your way through all the hype. Also, check out Web sites that I recommend in Chapter 21.

Part III

Turning to the Pros to Treat Your Type of Acne

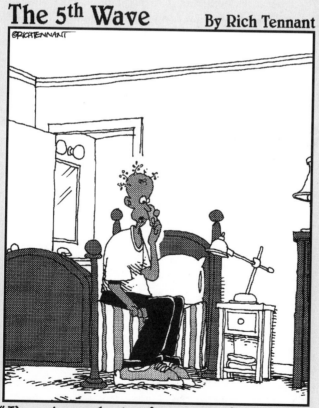

The 5th Wave   By Rich Tennant

"I'm using an herbal face cream for my skin. It's clearing up my acne, but now I'm growing alfalfa sprouts."

In this part . . .

I start off by helping you find a dermatologist or other medical professional to help you get your treatment underway. Then I clearly explain — in plain English — the many available treatment options that your doctor may recommend including topical medications, oral antibiotics, hormone therapy, Accutane, and lasers and lights. Within each discussion I highlight the preferred paths for teens, adults, and folks with dark skin. I also devote a chapter to exploring alternative and complementary therapies.

Chapter 8

Calling in the Experts

*A*cne can be tough to treat, especially on your own. If you're ready to consider a visit to the doctor (see the criteria I suggest for making this determination in Chapter 1), you've come to the right place. In this chapter, I look over the landscape of professional help that is available to manage your acne. Some general healthcare providers learn about treating acne as a part of their medical training, and your healthcare provider may be one of them. I fill you in on how to determine whether that's the case. If it's not, no problem: I explain how to find a *dermatologist,* a specialist who deals with all skin disorders.

I also give you some pointers about how to make the most of your experience in managing your acne with the experts. I give you the "ins and outs" of dealing with the first appointment, the paperwork, insurance issues, prescription refills, and all that other annoying, but necessary, stuff. And I tell you what to expect from your treatment and how to have a good working relationship with your acne doctor.

Establishing Basic Goals of Treatment

Whether you visit your primary care provider or a dermatologist, the basic aims in treating your acne are usually the following:

✔ To prevent your acne from scarring or to prevent further scarring if it has already been present.

✔ To decrease the physical and emotional pain of having acne lesions.

✔ Of course, to make you look better!

Discuss your goals with your healthcare provider. Get a feel for what to expect from your treatment, how long it will take, and what to do if it doesn't work out so well. In other words, try to get an idea about a best-case/worst-case scenario. Seeing a dermatologist or other skin-care specialist can be part of that plan.

Seeing Your Primary Healthcare Provider

Visiting your primary care provider (PCP) is a logical first step because, nowadays, more and more healthcare providers are learning about the treatment of diseases of the skin, including acne. They have more tools at their disposal to treat your acne than you do because they're often able to write prescriptions, if necessary, for medications. Plus, even if they aren't able to help you manage your acne, many insurance policies require that your PCP provide a referral for specialists, including dermatologists.

Working together to treat your acne

Your PCP may be a(n):

✔ **Pediatrician:** A physician who specializes in children.

✔ **Family practitioner:** A generalist who treats routine medical problems for people of all ages.

✔ **Internist:** A physician who specializes in treating medical conditions of adults.

Your PCP may also be a healthcare specialist who isn't a doctor:

✔ **Physician assistant (PA):** Physician assistants work under the supervision of a physician. They work interdependently with the understanding that the physician is available for consultation whenever needed. PAs can treat patients and, in most states, prescribe medicine.

> ✔ **Nurse practitioner (NP):** A nurse practitioner is a nurse with a
> graduate degree in advanced practice nursing. Some NPs
> work without physician supervision, and others work
> together with physicians as a joint healthcare team. Their
> range of practice and authority depends on state laws. For
> example, some states allow nurse practitioners to write pre-
> scriptions, and other states don't.

Some PAs and NPs are specifically trained in dermatology, and
some even specialize in areas such as acne. In fact, some PAs and
NPs may actually have more training in dermatology than pediatricians, internists, and family practitioners. An advantage to seeing a
physician assistant or nurse practitioner is that it may also
decrease the waiting time necessary for an appointment with a
busy physician.

But the next question is whether or not *your* PCP is able to manage
your acne. You should always find out about the experience your
PCP has had in treating acne. The best way to find out is by simply
asking him.

If you and your primary care provider decide to tackle your acne
together, she'll likely give you one or two topical medications to
apply to your skin. She may also give you certain oral antibiotics
that are effective in treating acne. (In Chapters 9 and 10, I give the
details about these agents that are used to treat acne.)

Be patient and give the medications a chance to work. Topical
medications can take weeks to months to show what they can do.
Keep in mind that medications should be used as directed or they
can't work nearly as well. Make a habit of taking or applying your
acne medicines like you make a habit of brushing your teeth.

It's not unusual for acne to last for many years, so ongoing treatment may be necessary.

It may come to pass that despite the best efforts of your PCP, your
expectations for improvement in your acne haven't been met.
You've been through the usual stuff — pills, creams, and lotions
that have been prescribed for you and you're not getting any
better, or not better enough to suit you. In this case, seeing a *dermatologist,* the expert in the management of this difficult and pesky
disorder, is an option to consider. Just about every case of acne
can be cleared up, but sometimes it takes a dermatologist's help.

What is a consultation?

A consultation is a meeting of two or more health professionals to discuss the diagnosis, prognosis, and treatment of your acne. The consultation is basically a request from your PCP to work with a dermatologist as a team to treat your acne.

The dermatologist sends a letter, an e-mail, or makes a telephone call to your PCP and describes what recommended treatment he feels would be best to treat your acne. Your PCP will then follow the consulting dermatologist's recommendations, and together they act as your acne skin-care team.

Ideally, theirs should be an "open-door" relationship that allows you to see the dermatologist again if things aren't working out.

Requesting a referral to see a specialist

If your health plan requires that referrals to specialists be authorized or approved by your PCP, who is often your best source, then you need to ask for the referral. However, if your health plan allows you to make appointments without a referral from your PCP, your PCP is still an excellent source for helping you to identify a qualified professional in your community (see "Finding the Right Dermatologist for You," later in this chapter).

You can enter into a specialist's care via a referral in a number of different ways, but in most cases, your specialized care typically falls into two categories:

- **For a consultation:** In some cases, your PCP may prefer to have you obtain a dermatology *consultation,* which means that the specialist will evaluate you and make recommendations for further care, and then send you back to your PCP for continuing treatment. For more on what to expect from a consultation, see the sidebar "What is a consultation?"

- **For ongoing treatment:** In this situation, your PCP requests that your acne-related care remain in the hands of the specialist. You would still continue to see your PCP for routine things like illnesses and injuries, but your specialist will handle all things related to your acne.

In either case, the medical records of your care to date should be sent or brought by you to the dermatology specialist to review so that any relevant medical information such as past medications and therapies will be available to her.

Finding the Right Dermatologist for You

All dermatologists aren't created equal. Some are very talented and up-to-the-minute on the latest knowledge for treating your acne, while others may lag in their capabilities. Start by asking your regular PCP for the person who might best treat your acne. You may want to ask him whom he would send a member of his own family to if they had acne.

A dermatologist must have a degree in medicine, either as a Medical Doctor (MD) or a Doctor of Osteopathic Medicine (DO). Dermatologists first go to medical school and then to a residency program for their specialized training. They're experts in the diagnosis and treatment of diseases of the skin (including hair and nails) in both pediatric and adult patients.

Depending on the doctor's specialty and interest, a dermatologist may also receive very specialized training in one or more of the following procedures (some of which I cover in Chapters 14 and 16):

- The use of lasers and other special light delivery systems to help treat acne
- Surgical corrective resurfacing procedures to reduce acne scars
- Various cosmetic techniques such as Botox and "filler" injections to improve the appearance of the face

In the following two sections, I tell you how to go about seeing a dermatologist, a PA, or an NP and what to do when you get there. From here on out, I refer to all of those professionals as dermatologists. After you put together a list of prospective dermatologists, call each office and ask if the doctor accepts your health insurance plan. If the doctor isn't covered by your plan, ask yourself if you're prepared to pay any extra costs.

Using networking techniques

In addition to checking in with your PCP, you could also locate a specialist on your own by asking your friends, family, or other members of your community who have been satisfactorily treated by a particular dermatologist. Don't be shy. If you know someone who had acne and now shows improvement, ask her how she did it. She'll likely be thrilled you noticed and happy to share the info.

If your house needed a renovation, you'd likely ask for references about any contractor that you might consider. The same holds true for anyone who is going to be responsible for your skin, the "house" you live in.

Checking in with professional associations

The American Academy of Dermatology is the largest dermatologic association in the United States. Their Web site (www.aad.org) can help you locate a dermatologist in your area. This site can also provide biographical information about many academy member dermatologists, including their education, specialized training, office hours, and whether they accept your health insurance plan. You can also find detailed maps showing how to get to their offices. You can also call or write to the American Academy of Dermatology, 930 E. Woodfield Road, Schaumburg, Illinois, 60173-4927; 847-330-0230.

You can find out whether the doctor you're interested in is board certified in dermatology. "Certified" means that she has completed a training program in the specialty of dermatology and has passed an exam, or "board," that assesses her knowledge, skills, and experience to provide quality patient care in that specialty. That means that all the training and tests have been met by the doctor and approved by the American Academy of Dermatology.

I would certainly recommend that you look for a dermatologist who is board certified.

Many dermatologists have teaching positions at academic centers such as major hospitals and medical or osteopathy schools. You can check out their credentials and academic positions online or by asking your local public or university reference librarian to help you.

Looking at your insurance directory

You know that list of names that came in the mail or that were given to you when you signed up with your HMO or other health insurance company? It contains a list of specialists who are in their *network of providers,* which means the doctor has been approved by your HMO or insurance company. An advantage to using an in-network specialist is that most insurers check out the providers on that list and hold them to high standards.

Moreover, if you go to a specialist who is on this approved list of providers, most of the medical bill will be covered by your insurer. Who doesn't want that?

If someone you wish to see isn't on that recommended list, it doesn't always mean that the specialist isn't up to snuff. In fact, it may be worth your while to go out of network to find the right person for you; however, it will likely cost you more money to do so.

Check with your insurance company to see whether they have an online directory. Typically, the directory doesn't include recommendations, per se. But you can search their directory based on specific criteria, like distance from a location (like your home or child's school) or office hours. Often you can click to find a map directly to the dermatologist's office and get the phone number to make an appointment right away.

Perusing the phone book and advertisements

Believe it or not, the phone book can help you with your choice. Specifically, it can help you choose:

- ✔ **A dermatologist that's close to your home or your child's school.** That makes sense.

- ✔ **A male or female.** You can then decide who you or your child would be most comfortable with.

- ✔ **One that may speak your language or has translation available to you if you don't speak English.** You could call to find out.

But remember, the bigger ad isn't always better.

Unfortunately, the late 1970s and early 1980s saw the removal of legal restrictions against advertising by those in the legal and medical professions. I advise you to distrust a doctor who advertises via large billboards, television, newspapers, gigantic yellow page ads, or subways. Some of these doctors may start treating their patients as customers, rather than as patients. I also strongly advise you to avoid skin-care spas that advertise laundry lists of treatments that they offer. I've seen an add that lists "laser treatment for acne scars, male breast reduction, breast enlargement for women, leg vein removal, buttock enlargement, buttock reduction, cosmetic skin surgery, broken blood vessels, microdermabrasion, chemical peels, laser lunchtime super peels, collagen/Botox treatments, hair restoration, laser hair removal, body contouring, liposuction." And last but not least, in smaller print, "acne, eczema, skin cancer screening, warts, mole removal, and rashes." And maybe they can check your car's tire pressure and oil while you're there.

Going to the Dermatologist for the First Visit

Whether the person you're seeing is a dermatologist, a physician assistant, or a nurse practitioner, it's a good idea to come prepared for your first visit.

Taking stock of your medical history

Before you walk out the door for your first appointment, review your medical history. Be prepared to tell the dermatologist what medications you take and what medical problems you have that, unknown to you, might play a role in your having acne or the treatment your doctor recommends.

Here are a few things your dermatologist may want to know:

- ✔ **Allergies:** Do you have any allergies to medications?
- ✔ **Other skin conditions:** Do you have a history of *eczema* (an itchy, inflammatory skin problem that's often hereditary and makes your skin very sensitive) or *contact dermatitis* (an allergic reaction or an irritant response to things that have touched your skin)? These problems can be important because they can make your skin more vulnerable to some of the topical treatments that are used to treat acne.

✔ **Medications, vitamins, and supplements:** Go through the items in your medicine cabinet. If you've recently swallowed it or rubbed it on, your doctor needs to know about it.

Bring the medications you've been using to treat your acne into the examining room. The actual tubes and bottles can help your dermatologist read all the ingredients (both active and inactive) in the medications and make more informed recommendations about where to go from here. If you don't have the empty tubes or bottles with you, write down the names of the medications and their dosages. If you've been using a medication, describe how long you have used it. Note any subjective information like: Was it irritating? Was it helpful?

Also make a list of non-acne products, such as birth control pills, vitamins, herbs, supplements, or other medication. Include the medications' names and dosages.

Preparing on the day of your visit

With your medical history in hand, there are a few additional steps you can take to make the most out of your first office visit:

✔ **Arrive 15 minutes early:** On your first visit to any healthcare provider's office, you're generally expected to fill out a form or two. Your new doctor will need — at a minimum — your name, address, medical history, drug allergies, and current medication. You will also need to provide information about your insurance coverage and how you expect to pay for your visits (such as with cash or credit card). Arrive at the office earlier than your scheduled appointment to take care of these issues.

✔ **Bring a parent:** If you're a minor, you should come in with a parent or guardian. A *minor* is a person under the legal age of consent, which is generally 18. Certain procedures or medications will require parental consent, so be sure, especially on that first visit, that an adult or legal guardian is present.

✔ **Bring your insurance card:** You will be asked for your insurance card or the card of the policy holder if coverage isn't in your name. If you don't have a card with you, you should at least know the name and date of birth of the cardholder.

✔ **Remove your makeup:** When you see a dermatologist and expect a careful examination of your face, you shouldn't be wearing makeup to conceal the reason you went there in the first place — your face!

I know from firsthand experience that trying to see through makeup is like trying to look out of a window when it's fogged up. The time involved in removing makeup in the examining room is better spent talking about your skin. So remove it before entering the examining room. If you hate appearing in public with a "naked" face, you can always reapply your makeup before you leave the office.

Meeting the doc

Your first visit with your doctor will involve a review of your medical history, focusing on the acne angle, an examination of your skin, and treatment recommendations. In addition to checking out your face, he may want to look at your chest and back because acne often occurs there as well. If your acne only involves your face, then there's no need for you to undress.

Communicating your personal acne story

The following are my typical first-visit questions about acne. You will undoubtedly be asked some or all of them. To ensure that you don't forget anything and that you and your doctor can make the best use of your time together, you may want to spend a few minutes thinking about these questions before the visit:

- How long have you had acne?
- Does it run in your family?
- Is there anyone in the family with severe scarring acne?
- What do you do to your skin each day — such as how many times a day do you wash your face?
- Are you applying or taking any medications?
- Do you pick at lesions?
- What seems to make it worse? Diet, exercise, medications, stress?
- What has been helpful? Sunlight, vacations, medications, winning the lottery?

And if you're a female, you'll also get these old standbys:

- Does it get worse before your period or at midcycle?
- Does makeup make it worse?
- Are your periods normal?

> ✔ Are you taking birth control pills and do they seem to help or worsen your acne?

> ✔ Have you noticed any unusual or excessive hair growth?

Understanding treatment recommendations

Based on a physical exam and your discussions with your dermatologist, she will recommend treatment options, which will likely include some sort of medication.

 Before leaving the examining room, make sure that all your questions have been answered. Your doctor is there to help you through the process, and questions are always welcome. You should know what to expect from your treatment and get a clear sense of its goals.

For example, make sure that your doctor has answered these questions, and if not, ask them:

> ✔ What are the side effects of the medication you are prescribing?

> ✔ How long will it take for the treatment to work?

> ✔ How long do you think my acne will last?

But my standard reply when a patient asks, "How long will it take for my face to clear up?" or "How long will I have acne?" is something like "Gee, my crystal ball is in the repair shop this week!"

Launching a Good Working Relationship

As in any ongoing relationship, especially if it may last for a long time, it's important to feel comfortable and have a sense of genuine rapport with your dermatologist. Key points in building this relationship include closely following your doctor's instructions, being patient, and feeling free to ask any questions that you may have.

Following instructions

You need to know some very specific information before you start popping those pills or rubbing the acne stuff on your face and body. And just like that manual that came with your new iPod or computer, the medication your doctor prescribed comes with instructions. If you're like me, you'll probably find them much easier to understand than your iPod or computer instructions.

Read those instructions! Both the instructions that come with each medication and any handouts given to you by your doctor or anyone on her staff contain valuable information about your treatment regimen. If you weren't given an instruction sheet or other handwritten directions regarding medications, call your doctor for any necessary clarification. (You could also read the info in Chapters 9 and 10, where I spell out in detail how to make the best of your medications.)

Being a "patient" patient

Some folks expect things to work overnight and don't give the medications a chance. Impatient patients are a very common problem! If you think the stuff your doctor gave you isn't working, often it's because you haven't given it enough time to really kick in. For example, benzoyl peroxide may take four to six weeks to really start working, and some topical medications such as the retinoids can take up to three months before they show their stuff. I go over the retinoids and benzoyl peroxides in much more detail in Chapter 9.

You see your face in the mirror every day. Your dermatologist only sees it when you come to the office for your appointments. The improvement, or lack thereof, will be much more evident to him.

Sure, you'll have some good days and bad days, but overall, it's important to stick with the routine and give it a real chance to work and judge the progress on a monthly rather than a daily basis. Rome wasn't built in a day and your acne won't disappear in a week!

Telephoning the dermatologist with questions

You, your healthcare provider, and her staff should view your acne treatment as a team effort. Like any good team, communication here is important, so don't hesitate to call the doctor's office with questions or concerns you have outside of your normal office visits.

Although office policies vary, the best time to call is in the morning after 9 a.m. when most offices are open. Many offices go "on service" during lunch hours and an answering machine (voicemail purgatory) or operator who isn't in the office may answer your call.

If you need to cancel or change an appointment, the receptionist can handle that information while you're on the phone. Other procedural-type queries may be fielded by members of the dermatologist's staff. And, if you have a fairly straightforward medical question, the receptionist may have a nurse call you back. But for more complicated situations and real "trouble shooting," ask to speak to the dermatologist or have him call you back directly.

Simply tell the person who answers, "I would like to speak to the doctor, and it's very important. Please have him call me back." Leave the times and phone numbers where you can be reached in the next 24 hours. (If it's not an emergency, don't say it is one!) The staff will then pull your chart and leave it for the doctor to review.

Here are some of the most common scenarios that call for a quick call to your dermatologist instead of sitting back and waiting for your next appointment, which may be three months away:

- ✔ **Your medication isn't working.** If a medication is causing you problems, not working, or for some reason you can't or won't use it, call the dermatologist about it — or if you're a kid ask your parent to call. *Don't wait.*

- ✔ **You forgot to ask certain questions during your appointment.** Call the dermatologist rather than waiting until your next appointment.

- ✔ **You need refills or you lost a prescription or medication.** Possibly you lost the actual prescription or you left the medication at your grandparents' house, at a camping trip site, or your dog ate it. Often the receptionist or nurse can take care of refills over the telephone. (If your dog ate your prescription, you may also need to call or visit the vet!)

  More often that not, when you call to ask for a refill, you'll find that there is a specific policy that is carefully followed. Most dermatologists, as well as many other healthcare providers, are more liberal when it comes to refilling topical medications. However, oral drugs carry greater risks and the policy regarding refilling them will necessarily be much stricter.

  Many dermatologists insist that you be seen in their office if more than a year has elapsed since your last office appointment before mailing you or telephoning your pharmacy for a refill. This is especially the case when the dermatologist isn't very familiar with your case and perhaps has only seen you on one or two occasions.

✔ **You need a different prescription.** Maybe you can't afford the prescription and need a generic substitute.

✔ **You lost information about the medication.** Maybe you forgot how often to take the pills or your PCP wants to give you a medicine for another condition and you want to know if that drug can be taken along with your acne medication.

✔ **You're concerned about side effects.** Maybe the stuff the dermatologist gave you smelled horrible, made your dog sick, upset your stomach, gave you a yeast infection, bleached your nice blouse, irritated your skin, or made you itch like crazy!

✔ **You need a referral.** For instance, you're moving to Albuquerque and you want the name of a dermatologist in that city.

Deciding to change dermatologists

You can switch dermatologists if you don't have a good communication with the dermatologist you're seeing or if you're not satisfied with the progress of your treatment. You or your parent might speak to the dermatologist about these issues and maybe give her and the medication(s) more time or another office visit or two before deciding to change doctors.

If you're still dissatisfied, ask your PCP for another referral, or repeat the measures that I talk about in the earlier section, "Finding the Right Dermatologist for You."

Chapter 9

Reviewing the Topical Tools at Your Dermatologist's Disposal

In This Chapter

▶ Choosing to treat your acne topically

▶ Evaluating a cornucopia of topical treatments

▶ Getting into generics

*Y*ou may have tried some over-the-counter products, flirted with various diets, or experimented with cosmetics, facials, and soaps. Maybe you've even watched a few TV infomercials and tried those products with unsatisfactory results. Well, it sounds like you're ready for a different approach. The good news is that doctors have a treasure trove of excellent topical tools they can use to treat any type of acne. In fact, for many people, topical preparations are the only treatment necessary.

In this chapter, I tell you all you need to know about the topical preparations available through a healthcare provider to treat your acne and how to use them effectively.

Before starting out on our acne treatment journey, there are three important points that you as an acne patient should be aware of:

✔ Six to eight weeks of treatment may be required before you see any significant improvement.

✔ Lesions on the back, chest, and shoulders respond more slowly to topical and oral treatment than do those on the face.

✔ Every patient is an individual, and as such your doctor is in the best position to tailor treatments to your needs. Always follow your doctor's recommendations.

Taking the Topical Route

The use of topicals offers many advantages over *oral therapy* (taking medications by mouth). The most obvious advantage is that your skin gets the direct application of medications and very few serious complications can result, whereas the oral route may lead to more severe side effects (such as those discussed in Chapter 10). In topical therapy, a *vehicle* (an inactive medium) "delivers" the *active ingredient* (the drug itself) to its intended target. The vehicle may be a cream, ointment, gel, lotion, or *solution* (an oil-free liquid, that's usually composed of water or alcohol).

 The solutions, gels, and lotions that contain active ingredients can also hitch a ride on convenient travel-friendly delivery systems, such as the *pledget* or *swab*. These are small absorbent pads, used to medicate the skin, that are made from cotton or wool. Just put them in your bag, backpack, or pocket, and away you go.

In the treatment of acne, the vehicle may be as important as the drug or drugs that it transports. A vehicle gives a product its texture and substance and can sometimes determine its strength and influence how effectively a drug gets absorbed. Check out Chapter 7 for more on the general principles of topical therapy.

 Different topical treatments for different forms of acne are determined by many factors, such as:

- Your skin type: dry, oily, combination, or normal
- The types of lesions you have: blackheads and whiteheads, papules and pustules, or both
- How long your lesions have been present
- Your past response to acne treatments and side effects that you've encountered
- Your tendency to develop scarring or disfiguring acne spots
- How much a treatment costs you and whether you can afford it

 The best product is one that works best for *you*. Topical treatment frequently involves a trial-and-error approach, beginning with those products that are known to be most effective, least expensive, and have the fewest side effects. As you find things that don't work, you and your doctor team up to remove them from your regimen and add different (and hopefully better-for-you) products. That's why it's important for you to have a continuing dialog with your dermatologist in order to come up with the right product or combination of products for you to apply.

Sometimes your dermatologist may choose to combine a drying product (most acne products are), together with a moisturizing product in order to make the drying product less irritating.

Opening Up the Tool Chest

Topical acne therapy aims to counter several of the major factors that cause acne:

- ✔ Blocked hair follicles
- ✔ Growth of the acne causing bacteria, *P. acnes*
- ✔ Inflammation

Oral therapy is required to tackle the other important acne causing factors, such as:

- ✔ Increased hormone production
- ✔ Excess sebum (oil) production

I describe these factors in detail (including the fancy medical terms involved with each of them) in Chapter 3.

Topical treatment is sufficient for most people who have acne, but oral reinforcements are generally a must if you have more extensive, deep, or scarring acne with nodules and cysts. Chapter 10 is where you can find information about the oral weapons. The following sections offer a wide range of topical treatments for your acne. Keep in mind that one size doesn't fit all and fitting the proper medication to your skin sometimes takes trying different ones for a while.

Most dermatologists agree that the *combination therapy* — the use of topical retinoids and topical or oral antibiotics or antibacterials such as benzoyl peroxide — reduces both inflammatory and non-inflammatory lesions more rapidly and to a greater degree than can be effected with any of these agents alone.

Reviewing topical retinoids

Most dermatologists consider topical retinoids to be the mainstay of acne therapy. They're often the first-line prescription treatment for acne and they're also utilized as long-term maintenance for almost every acne patient. Retinoids are, far and above, the drugs of choice in people who have *comedonal* (blackhead and whitehead) acne, but they're also effective at fighting inflammatory lesions, so chances are that your dermatologist will start you off with one of these.

Retinoids are medications that are derived from vitamin A. Retinoids are *comedolytic,* which means that they work by making the skin shed more easily so that follicular plugs don't build up and form blackheads and whiteheads. In addition to helping you shed your skin, retinoids

- ✔ Indirectly limit the formation of inflammatory lesions by preventing comedones. After all, if comedones don't ever form, they can't become big, inflamed pustules and papules.

- ✔ Appear to discourage *P. acnes* (the bacterial invaders associated with acne) growth.

- ✔ Promote the shedding of skin, which enhances the penetration of other topical anti-acne agents.

- ✔ Help to "plump up" the skin and make enlarged pores (*follicular prominence,* in dermatologist speak) less obvious.

Several brand-name topical retinoids, as well as generic preparations, are on the market (check out Table 9-1 for information on which brand-name retinoids contain which active ingredient, and read the sidebar in this chapter to get a handle on what a "branded generic" is). Many studies have been performed on the topical retinoids and the results don't clearly favor the use of one preparation over another. Individuals vary in their response to these agents and possible side effects, so you and your doctor will work together to find the best prescription for you.

Generic versus "branded generic" drugs

It's a tricky business trying to find cheaper drugs. When a famous drug such as Retin-A has its patent expire, it can then become a generic (unbranded) drug. As an example, once a brand becomes generic, the original company often ceases to promote or support it. Sometimes this can be a real benefit because the generic version tends to be considerably cheaper. Hurray!

But, after a while, some generic companies come along and obtain approval from the FDA to manufacture the drug and they put the original brand name on it. When that happens, the *branded generic* price becomes higher than the generic price because of the cost of marketing.

Sounds like double speak, a kind of contradiction in terms, doesn't it? The bottom line is try to be an educated consumer. Read labels and compare prices! To find an updated list of generic and branded generic drugs, go to: www.wellmark.com/drugformulary/df_main.asp.

Table 9-1	The Topical Retinoids		
Brand Name	**Generic Name**	**Delivery**	**Strengths**
Retin-A* (Branded generic)	Tretinoin	Cream, solution	0.025% 0.05% 0.1% 0.5%
Retin-A* (Branded generic)	Tretinoin	Gel	0.01% 0.025%
Retin-A Micro	Tretinoin	Microsphere gel	0.1%
Avita*	Tretinoin	Cream, gel	0.025%
Differin	Adapalene	Cream, gel, solution, and pledgets	0.1%
Tazorac	Tazarotene	Cream, gel	0.05% 0.1%

*Apply only at bedtime

Because of the known *teratogenic effects* (anything which produces nonheritable birth defects) of *oral* vitamin A, the use of topical retinoids in pregnancy has been an issue of concern. Although no studies have shown them to cause any birth defects, it is recommended that these drugs *should not* be used during pregnancy or breastfeeding.

Applying retinoids like a pro

Topical retinoids are applied in small, thin, pea-sized amounts to clean, dry skin once a day in the morning or at bedtime. They should be applied to all affected areas as well as to places that are acne-prone. Retin-A (not Retin-A Micro) and Avita, which tend to degrade in sunlight, should be applied only at bedtime. Talk with your doctor about the best time to apply Retin-A Micro, Differin, and Tazorac.

Dermatologists often start treatments with a lower strength preparation; in time, your doctor may prescribe higher concentrations of the active ingredient, if necessary, depending on your ability to tolerate them.

Within six to eight weeks, you should notice improvement if you have been using your product continuously. Maximal improvement most often occurs by three to four months.

Despite the common misconception, acne does not flare in the first few weeks of treatment; rather, the "flare" is due to irritation from the retinoid or from the natural progression of your acne, so try to "ride it through" unless the irritation is really severe — at which point you should call your dermatologist or healthcare provider.

It's not uncommon for retinoids to be used improperly and discarded before they have a real chance to work. Make sure you get both verbal and written directions from your doctor to make sure that you use your products correctly.

Dealing with side effects

All retinoids can cause some skin irritation during the first few weeks of use. You may have some discomfort, such as stinging or burning, and sometimes may experience mild redness and scaling of your skin. These reactions are to be expected, and they're an indication that the retinoid is working. After several weeks, your skin generally gets used to the medication and the discomfort eases.

A common belief is that retinoids dry the skin. But they're actually sloughing off dead skin cells.

If you have a sensitivity to the retinoid you were prescribed, you can take a number of steps to help ease the irritation:

- ✔ **Build up a tolerance:** Start off by using the retinoid every other day, or even less frequently, until you get used to it.

  If you have extremely sensitive skin, try applying the retinoid for short periods of time, such as leaving it on for a few minutes and then washing it off. You can put it on for as little as two to five minutes. This tends to make it more tolerable and the medicine still has positive effects as long as you stick with it. As your skin becomes accustomed to the retinoid, you can gradually increase the frequency of application and how long you leave it on. Eventually you may be able to apply it every day and leave it on all day or overnight.

- ✔ **Avoid irritating OTC products:** Make sure that you're not also using an over-the-counter product that contains salicylic acid, retinols, or other possible irritants.

- ✔ **Ask your doctor to prescribe a cream or a weaker concentration of the medicine.** Creams are the least irritating delivery vehicle. The concentration of the agent affects the degree of irritation.

- ✔ **Use a moisturizer:** If you get dry and scaly, apply a moisturizer generously in the morning. The moisturizer should be applied *over* any medication you apply at night or in the

morning. (If you also use a sunscreen, apply it over the moisturizer.) Effective moisturizers include Oil of Olay, Nivea Ultra
Moisturizing Creme, and Eucerin creams. Use only emollient,
non-irritating cleansers to wash your face when you're using a
topical retinoid.

Retinoids may produce sun sensitivity. A common misconception
is that tretinoin shouldn't be used during the summertime, during
sunny weather, or in tropical climates. Retinoids can make you
somewhat more susceptible to sunburn, however, this problem
eases after the drug has been used for a month or two. Retinoids
can be applied at any time of year in any geographic region.

If you're using a retinoid in sunny conditions, particularly if you
have fair skin, just take simple sun-protective measures, such as
avoiding the midday sun, applying a broad-spectrum sunscreen or
sunblock (over the medication), and wearing a protective cap or
hat. Applying them at bedtime is added insurance against your
having problems with sun exposure the next day.

Enhancing retinoid treatment

Removal of comedones can also help to treat your acne and speed
up improvement. Your dermatologist may perform *acne surgery*
with a *comedo extractor,* a small instrument that mechanically
removes comedones. Comedo removal can be a useful adjunct to
topical therapy when your blackheads and whiteheads are somewhat resistant to topical retinoids.

Acne surgery is a *noninvasive surgery,* meaning that the blackheads
and whiteheads are simply popped or squeezed out with the extractor. The *extractor* is a special instrument that minimizes skin injury.
A round loop extractor is used to apply uniform smooth pressure to
dislodge the material. Lesions that offer resistance are loosened by
inserting a pointed instrument to carefully expose the contents.

Pretreatment with a topical retinoid for four to six weeks often
facilitates the procedure because it helps open up your pores.
Comedo extraction is performed less commonly nowadays since
the arrival of topical retinoids.

Comedo extraction is often performed successfully by aestheticians as part of a facial. An experienced technician may remove
your blackheads and whiteheads with tissue paper or with another
instrument.

An improperly trained technician may also try to squeeze out your
red papules which can result in persistent redness and even scarring.

Turning to topical antibiotics

Because retinoids may be more difficult for you to tolerate and can take a long time to work, your dermatologist may elect to treat your inflammatory lesions (papules and pustules) first with oral or topical antibiotics. They work much faster than the retinoids. So if you're in a hurry to look better, the quicker response can be a helpful incentive for you to continue therapy.

Clindamycin and *erythromycin* are the two most commonly used topical antibiotics for the management of inflammatory acne. Dermatologists consider them to be equally effective. They can be used alone or in combination with benzoyl peroxide and/or oral antibiotics (see Chapter 10 for more on oral antibiotics) to treat acne as well as rosacea, perioral dermatitis, shaving bumps, and other acnelike conditions. (I discuss these conditions in Chapters 18 and 19.)

 Topical antibiotics directly kill *P. acnes*. In addition to their antibacterial action, these drugs have an anti-inflammatory action that helps to clear inflammatory acne lesions. Through their bacterial killing ability, they also appear to have a mild indirect blocking effect on the formation of blackheads and whiteheads (known by the fancy medical name of *comedogenesis*). Check out more about how blackheads and whiteheads form in Chapter 3. Topical antibiotics are available in creams, ointments, gels, solutions, and lotions.

This variety allows your dermatologist or healthcare provider to prescribe according to your skin type or preference. Many prescription topical antibiotics are available, as you can see in Table 9-2. Some erythromycin and clindamycin products have become available as generics, while other have become branded generics. (See the sidebar on branded generics.)

Table 9-2	Topical Antibiotics		
Brand Name	*Generic Name*	*Delivery*	*Strengths*
(Branded generics)*	Erythromycin	Solution, gel, lotion, swabs	2%
A/T/S	Erythromycin	Solution, gel	2%
Theramycin Z**	Erythromycin	Solution	2%
Akne-Mycin	Erythromycin	Ointment	2%
Erycette	Erythromycin	Pledgets	2%
Staticin	Erythromycin	Solution	1.5 %

Brand Name	Generic Name	Delivery	Strengths
(Branded generics)*	Clindamycin	Solution, gel, lotion, pledgets	1%
Cleocin T	Clindamycin	Solution, gel, lotion, pledgets	1%
ClindaMax	Clindamycin	Gel, lotion	1%
Clindets	Clindamycin	Pledgets	1%

* There are numerous branded generics of these agents
**Contains zinc

Applying antibiotics for the best results

Topical antibiotics are applied once or twice daily, in a thin layer on all of the acne-prone areas to clean, dry skin. In four to six weeks, you should see a decrease in the size of inflammatory acne lesions. The therapeutic response tends to be more effective when the topical antibiotic is combined with benzoyl peroxide (see "Combining benzoyl peroxide with topical antibiotics," later in this chapter).

Topical antibiotics may promote the appearance of resistant strains of *P. acnes*. Resistance is diminished by combining them with or using them in conjunction with benzoyl peroxide (see the "Combining benzoyl peroxide with topical antibiotics" section).

Dealing with side effects

Mild side effects such as redness, skin irritation, and scaling are associated with use of these drugs, but most people tolerate topical antibiotics well.

If you have a skin condition known as eczema, you may have extremely sensitive skin. Irritation and burning may be associated with applying certain topical antibiotic preparations. This may be avoided if you're prescribed an ointment-based erythromycin such as Akne-Mycin or clindamycin in a lotion preparation.

Combining benzoyl peroxide with topical antibiotics

Benzoyl peroxide is the mainstay of over-the-counter acne treatment (and I provide a full rundown of these benzoyl peroxide products in Chapter 7, along with all the other OTC acne medications). In addition to using benzoyl peroxide alone to treat your mild acne, benzoyl peroxide is also often used in conjunction with topical or systemic antibiotics. This treatment option is referred to as *combination therapy*. In fact, combination therapy is used to treat most cases of acne because it's caused by a combinations of factors. I explain these factors in Chapter 3.

Combination therapy can refer to using combination products, such as those in Benzamycin, Duac, or BenzaClin, or by using them in addition to a topical retinoid and an oral antibiotic, for example. By using drugs that have different means and modes of activity, your acne is attacked on many fronts.

Combining benzoyl peroxide with erythromycin or clindamycin has the following advantages:

✔ In contrast to topical antibiotics used alone, adding benzoyl peroxide to the mixture prevents *P. acnes* from becoming resistant to them.

✔ The combination also appears to have a *synergistic effect* (the combination works better than either agent used alone).

Table 9-3 tells you the names of these preparations.

Table 9-3	Combination Benzoyl Peroxide with Topical Antibiotics	
Brand Name	**Generic Name/Strengths**	**Delivery**
Benzamycin* (Branded generic)	5% benzoyl peroxide 3% erythromycin	Gel
Benzamycin Pak (Foil pouches)	5% benzoyl peroxide 3% erythromycin	Gel
BenzaClin Topical Gel**	5% benzoyl peroxide 1% clindamycin	Gel
Duac Gel	5% benzoyl peroxide 1% clindamycin	Gel

* Refrigeration is necessary to maintain potency
** Sometimes these agents come unmixed and the pharmacist or you must combine the clindamycin or erythromycin powder with the benzoyl peroxide gel.

If you're on the go — for instance traveling or camping, or you're a teen that splits time between two homes — the Benzamycin Pak comes in foil pouches, which are easier to deal with.

If you're looking to save some money on your combination acne treatments, talk to your doctor about using a prescription for a generic topical antibiotic such as clindamycin or erythromycin lotion along with an over-the-counter benzoyl peroxide. Use them one on top of the other.

How to apply them

Before applying medicine to affected areas, wash your skin gently, rinse with warm water, and pat dry. (If you'd like to check out some face-washing tips, see Chapter 2.) Apply the gels in small, pea-sized amounts once or twice a day or as directed by your doctor, in the morning or at bedtime to all of your acne-prone areas.

When used alone, the benzoyl peroxide/antibiotic combination takes about four to six weeks to show significant improvement. Once-a-day applications are usually sufficient and allow for the application of other topicals such as retinoids, if they are required, at another time of day.

If you have blackheads and whiteheads (comedones), a comedolytic agent such as a topical retinoid may be prescribed for you to apply at a different time of day. To minimize irritation, try alternating the products daily for two weeks until you adapt to using them both daily.

Side effects

You can expect the same dry skin and skin irritation that are the most common side effects for benzoyl peroxide, plus the slight chance of mild irritation from the topical antibiotics. Side effects may include dry skin, itching, peeling, redness, and possibly a contact dermatitis from the sensitivity to the benzoyl peroxide. This condition is described in Chapter 7.

To combat excessive dryness, apply a moisturizer generously in the morning. (Check out the section "Reviewing topical retinoids," earlier in this chapter, for the names of some good moisturizers.) If you apply medication in the morning, the moisturizer should be applied *over* the medicated gels so that you don't block them from doing their job.

As with the topical retinoids, use only emollient, non-irritating cleansers to wash your face when you're using these preparations.

If you find that the combination products are too irritating (that's usually due to the benzoyl peroxide in them), you might try an over-the-counter water-based benzoyl peroxide preparation such as Neutrogena On-the-Spot Acne Treatment, or a benzoyl peroxide soap bar such as Fostex 10% BPO Wash. There are also prescription benzoyl peroxide washes such as Zoderm and Triaz Cleansers.

All of these products may be left on the skin for 5 minutes and then rinsed off. Afterward, a topical antibiotic preparation such as clindamycin or erythromycin can be applied. That way, you still can get the benzoyl peroxide effect and hopefully avoid the irritation.

Looking at other topicals

Newer agents, such as azelaic acid, and older preparations that contain sulfur and sodium sulfacetamide are used as alternatives or add-ons to retinoids, benzoyl peroxide, and benzoyl peroxide/antibiotic preparations. They're the second line of defense when the first team isn't doing so well or, more commonly, isn't tolerated.

Azelaic acid

For those of you who want to go a more "natural route," azelaic acid might be right up your alley. Azelaic acid is a naturally occurring acid found in grains like wheat, rye, and barley. Azelaic acid has been shown to possess:

✔ Antibacterial activity against *P. acnes*

✔ A mild anti-inflammatory effect

✔ A minor reduction on comedone (blackheads and whitehead) formation

Azelaic acid can be found in 20 percent creams under the brand names Azelex or Finevin. Apply it in small, pea-sized amounts once or twice a day to a clean, dry face to all acne-prone areas.

Most people start to see improvement in their acne within four to six weeks. It is tolerated fairly well; however, some people experience mild side effects such as redness and scaling.

 Because azelaic acid decreases pigmentation, it should be used with some caution in patients with darker complexions. On the other hand, this side effect can be an added benefit in people of color in the treatment of dark spots that often occur when their acne heals. (See Chapter 12 where I discuss acne in Asian, African, Afro-Caribbean, and African-American skin.)

Topical sulfacetamide/sulfur combinations

The combination of sulfacetamide and sulfur can be effective in the treatment of inflammatory skin lesions without the unpleasant side effects (primarily a rotten egg odor) that occur with sulfur preparations alone. They're less effective than retinoids, benzoyl peroxide, and benzoyl-peroxide-and-antibiotic combinations, but as with azelaic acid, they're sometimes useful as adjunctive therapy for the inflammatory component of acne as well as for rosacea (see Chapter 18).

Sulfacetamide/sulfur combinations are available as lotions, creams, and washes. You can find a host of products that contain sodium sulfacetamide 10 percent and sulfur 5 percent, such as Rosula, Rosac, Rosanil, Nicosyn, and Novacet, to name a few. Rosac also contains a sunscreen. In general, apply these products twice a day on clean dry skin to all acne-prone areas.

Some of these preparations have color tinting in them so that they can serve as a cosmetic cover-up to hide the redness of acne. Sulfacet-R is one of them. This medicine comes with a color blender that allows you to change the tint of the lotion to match your skin color.

In my experience, these products have a marginal utility and appear to have less anti-inflammatory effect than the topical anti-biotics I describe in this chapter. If you use them, expect a slower, and less effective, response than you get with other treatments. Mild stinging and redness may occur with these products.

Going Generic

Did you know that when you have a prescription to be filled, you may have a choice between filling it with a brand-name drug or a generic drug? *Generic* drugs are pharmaceuticals that are essentially similar to an original product that had been on the market for years.

The active ingredients in the original product are protected by a patent for a specific period of time. When a patent expires, a generic drug company introduces a copycat version of the original drug. Because the original drug has been a proven commodity, the generic versions are expected to work just as well as the originals.

Generic medications are

✔ **Generally 30 to 60 percent less expensive than the equivalent brand-name product.** Help control health insurance costs for yourself and everybody else by asking for generic drugs when possible. Ask your doctor to indicate on the prescription that *substitution is permitted* if you want a generic prescription. When you get to the pharmacy, ask if a generic version of your drug is available and ask the pharmacist to substitute the generic for the brand-name drug unless your doctor has written on the prescription that *no substitution* can be made.

Topicals in the pipeline

Topical Atrisone is a new gel preparation that contains dapsone (avlosulfon). Studies have indicated that topical dapsone reduces both inflammatory and non-inflammatory acne lesions. At this point, it's unclear how it will rate against our other acne drugs. As of this printing, patients using gels that contain dapsone have to be screened by a blood test to see whether they are predisposed to a certain type of anemia that can be associated with oral dapsone. Further cllinical trials are planned in hopes of having this testing requirement lifted

Clindamycin and tretinoin in combination is now in the investigational phase as of this printing. This treatment may prove to be an excellent combination of two very effective drugs. But why wait? You can do it yourself now — with prescriptions from your doctor, of course — and make your own combination clindamycin and tretinoin. A generic retinoid and generic topical antibiotic can be combined in the same manner as I describe in the section earlier, "Combining benzoyl peroxide with topical antibiotics." Just layer the topical retinoid over a generic clindamycin or erythromycin lotion.

- ✔ **Most often just as effective even though they cost less.** Applicants for generic drug approval must scientifically demonstrate that their product is *bioequivalent* (meaning that it performs in the same manner) to the brand-name drug.

- ✔ **Made of the same active ingredient or ingredients and the same strength as the brand name.** Bioequivalent medications contain the same active ingredients and are subject to the same Food and Drug Administration (FDA) standards for quality, strength, safety, potency, and purity as their brand-name counterparts. They must also produce the same effect on the body as the brand-name counterpart.

The TV infomercial and Internet acne products marketed as "total acne treatment systems" are now available over the counter as generic "house brands." They're sitting on the shelves of many of your local stores at a great savings.

Some generics don't have the same effectiveness as the well-known brand. If you aren't doing well on a generic, you might want to ask for the brand-name version. Even though generics still contain the same active ingredient as the original branded drug, their vehicles may be sub par and there may be instances when they act somewhat differently on or in your body. Talk about it with your doctor.

For more information about generic drugs, you can go to the following Web site: www.fda.gov/cder/ogd/index.htm.

Chapter 10

Taking the Oral Antibiotic Route

*I*f your acne isn't responding to topical treatments, then oral therapy is probably the next step. This chapter looks at the primary oral agents used to treat acne: antibiotics. We sometimes treat acne in women with hormones. I cover that therapy in Chapter 11. And the most powerful acne drug of all, Accutane, is discussed separately in Chapter 13. These oral agents are usually prescribed to be used in combination with the topical drugs you may have already been applying.

In this chapter, I give you the scoop on the advantages and disadvantages to the major acne-fighting oral antibiotics. I help you understand the dosing strategies and give you the tips to discuss with your doctor for using the medication to get the best results for you. (You can only get these drugs with a prescription from your doctor.) And finally, I show you where to get help if you're having trouble with your oral medications.

Calling In the Reinforcements

Oral antibiotics are used in the management of moderate to severe acne. As with the topical antibiotics discussed in Chapter 9, oral antibiotics work on acne by virtue of their antibacterial and anti-inflammatory effects.

Compared with topical therapy, oral therapy has a more rapid onset of action and works faster to improve your acne. Commonly, though, multiple medications are combined for the most effective treatment of acne. So in most cases, patients use more than one medication at any given time. By using drugs that have different means and modes of activity — for example, by taking oral antibiotics *and* applying a topical treatment — you attack your acne on several fronts. In designing your treatment regimen, your doctor can choose combinations of different classes of drugs that work on different targets, based on the severity of your acne and the possible side effects of the medication.

Being prescribed oral medications is not a message that you should stop applying topical medications! Make sure you go over your full medication regimen with your doctor before you leave her office. If you have questions later after you leave, call back to clarify.

Deciding it's time for oral antibiotics

Your doctor may decide to add oral antibiotic therapy to your topical therapy because the topical medications are

- ✔ Working too slowly
- ✔ Not doing the job well enough to suit you
- ✔ Not working at all

Or:

- ✔ Your acne is scarring
- ✔ You have moderate to severe inflammatory lesions
- ✔ Your lesions are widespread, even on your chest and your back
- ✔ Your prom is coming up next month
- ✔ You experience big swings in your acne that are related to your period (if you're female, of course)
- ✔ You're becoming depressed

Addressing some common concerns

Whenever oral drugs are taken, the potential dangers — including side effects, drug allergy, drug resistance, drug intolerance, drug interactions, and fetal exposure in women who are or may become pregnant — must be carefully considered.

A risk-benefit assessment is particularly important whenever a *benign* (non-life-threatening) condition such as acne is being treated. That means that you should ask your doctor about the advantages of taking an oral medication versus the disadvantages (such as possible scarring) of not taking it. Ask about the possible side effects — the risks — and what positive things you might expect — the benefits — if you take the drug.

Antibiotics, both topical and oral, have been central to the treatment of acne for many years. However, public health concerns about their widespread use has increased in recent years due to a number of issues:

✔ **Bacterial resistance:** *Resistance* means that a medicine no longer works, or becomes less effective, because the bacteria change (mutate) and no longer respond to the drug that is trying to kill or suppress them. No matter how many new antibiotics we come up with to fight *P. acnes,* the bacterium seems to find a way to outwit us and become resistant to our latest weapons. It's like trying to fight computer viruses that find ways to adapt to ever-changing methods we use to destroy them.

Despite the well-founded concerns about creating bacterial resistance, these drugs have a long track record of safety. They're effective, efficient treatments for many people who have acne as well as acnelike disorders, such as rosacea (see Chapter 18).

✔ **Purported links between oral antibiotics and breast cancer:** A well-publicized study suggested that the long-term use of antibiotics is associated with an increased risk of developing breast cancer. The study indicated that the risk was dependent on the cumulative dose and the amount of time a woman was taking antibiotics. The study had many flaws and never came to the conclusion that there was a direct causal link between antibiotics and breast cancer.

✔ **Antibiotics' influence on the efficacy of birth control pills:** Studies have shown that none of the antibiotics used commonly to treat acne interfered with the efficacy of oral contraceptives (see Chapter 11). But a woman can get pregnant while on any brand of birth control pill, whether taking antibiotics or not.

A recent study has suggested that the ingestion of oral antibiotics as well as the use of topical antibiotics in the treatment of acne *may* be associated with an increased risk of infectious respiratory diseases such as strep throat infections.

The best take-home message for you is that you should try your best to limit long-term use of antibiotics as much as possible until further studies and more data become available.

Worry about the safety of long-term oral medications has lead to a recent interest in the use of physical treatments such as lasers and other special light therapies to treat acne. Chapter 14 reviews some of these innovative procedures. For more information on how you and your doctor can work together to reduce antibiotic use, see the section "Surveying Strategies to Reduce Antibiotic Use," later in this chapter.

Tetracyclines: The First Team

The tetracyclines are the workhorses in oral acne therapy. They're the first-line oral antibiotic drugs of choice in the management of moderate to severe acne.

The tetracycline preparations inhibit the growth of *P. acnes* by going right to your sebaceous glands to attack the bacteria. They're *bacteriostatic* antibiotics, which means that they inhibit the growth of bacteria rather than kill them. In addition, they have an anti-inflammatory action that is equally important in the treatment of patients with papules and pustules.

There are three types of tetracyclines:

- ✔ "Plain" (generic) tetracycline
- ✔ Minocycline
- ✔ Doxycycline

Improvement of acne is usually noticeable in a matter of a few weeks or less with all of these tetracyclines. This response varies and depends on the severity of your acne; however, you may see the papules and pustules begin to flatten and disappear, and new ones should stop popping up. Tetracyclines may be tapered when this improvement persists. The decision about when and if to taper your dosage will be up to you and your doctor to decide. Often they have to be continued for long stretches of time — sometimes even for years.

Reviewing warnings, risks, and side effects of tetracyclines

Despite the low risk of side effects from tetracyclines, before taking the drugs, you should know a few things.

Because patients frequently use anti-acne oral antibiotics on a long-term basis (in some instances, for years), many people are understandably concerned about possible consequences. Studies have indicated that routine laboratory supervision of healthy young people given long-term tetracycline therapy isn't necessary. In a nutshell, in most cases, you don't need regular blood tests done while taking these antibiotics.

When treatment extends for more than one to two years, however, some dermatologists recommend periodically monitoring certain blood tests. This is particularly important if you have a history of liver, kidney, or an autoimmune disease. In such cases, you should get them checked more often.

Damage to teeth and bones

One of the main side effects of tetracycline is staining the teeth of children. There are also risks to the teeth and bones of unborn babies and nursing children. You shouldn't take them if you are:

- ✔ **A child under 10 years of age:** The use of any of the tetracyclines during a child's tooth development (before the age of 10) may cause a permanent discoloration of the teeth.

- ✔ **A woman who is breastfeeding or pregnant:** If a tetracycline is taken during pregnancy or while breastfeeding, an infant's teeth can become discolored and there also may be a slowing down of the infant's bone growth. The discoloration of the baby teeth is due to calcification (hardening) of the teeth, which starts in the second trimester (after 12 weeks of pregnancy).

Tetracyclines may also temporarily stain the teeth of older patients, particularly those with orthodontic braces. When taking any one of the tetracyclines, you should practice good dental hygiene, including flossing.

Other side effects

Here are some other side effects that may occur when taking the tetracyclines:

✔ As with many other antibiotics, you may experience mild indigestion and abdominal upset. They can also cause more severe gastrointestinal irritation (inflammation of your esophagus or stomach).

✔ Rashes are uncommon, but when they appear, they can be severe.

✔ They can sometimes produce phototoxic reactions (an increased tendency to sunburn). This reaction is more likely to occur with doxycycline (see the section later in this chapter).

✔ If you have a history of vaginal yeast infections known as *candidal vulvovaginitis,* a broad-spectrum antibiotic such as a tetracycline or an erythromycin (see the "Second-Line Oral Antibiotics" section, later in the chapter) can permit such an infection to reappear. Candidal vulvovaginitis can also occur for the first time when using these antibiotics.

And use them cautiously if you have a personal or family history of lupus erythematosus (an autoimmune disease). And don't take them if you're allergic to any of the tetracyclines.

Tetracyclines also have the following very rare risks:

✔ Severe headaches due to increased pressure in the brain *(intracranial hypertension)* are seen very rarely. However, you can get "regular" headaches from the tetracyclines without developing this complication.

✔ A hivelike, hypersensitivity rash, which includes joint swelling.

✔ Drug-induced hepatitis with jaundice (yellowish discoloration of the whites of the eyes, skin, and mucous membranes), nausea, and dark urine.

If you develop any of the preceding symptoms, call your doctor immediately.

Taking generic ("plain") tetracycline

By "plain" tetracycline we doctors mean the original, generic, or "branded generic," tetracyclines. I list the available forms in Table 10-1.

Table 10-1	"Plain" Tetracyclines		
Brand Name	*Generic Name*	*Delivery*	*Common Starting Dosages*
[Generic]	Tetracycline	Capsule, tablet, syrup	250 or 500 mg, twice a day
Achromycin (Branded generic)	Tetracycline	Capsule, tablet, syrup	250 or 500 mg, twice a day
Sumycin (Branded generic)	Tetracycline	Capsule, tablet, syrup	250 or 500 mg, twice a day

"Plain" tetracyclines are the most cost-effective of the tetracyclines and are much less expensive than minocycline and doxycycline, both of which I describe later in this chapter. However, "plain" tetracycline isn't always as effective as these two drugs when it comes to treating your acne.

Tetracycline is given in dosages ranging from 250 milligrams twice a day to 500 milligrams twice a day. It is usually begun at a dose of 500 milligrams twice daily, although 250 milligrams twice daily may also be effective.

Plain tetracycline is taken with a full glass of water so it doesn't irritate your esophagus, which can be a really painful experience. Take it on an empty stomach. (Your stomach is empty one hour before or two hours after meals.) And finally, don't take it with dairy products such as milk or with products that contain iron, magnesium, zinc, or calcium, because these compounds may interfere with tetracycline's absorption from your stomach and make it less effective.

The dosage of the drug may be tapered as inflammation lessens (usually after six to eight weeks), but this will vary depending upon your individual response.

Taking minocycline

Minocycline is a very effective oral antibiotic for treating acne. It's also the most expensive. Minocycline is available in generic formulations and is sold under several brand names, including those I list in Table 10-2.

Table 10-2		The Minocyclines	
Brand Name	*Generic Name*	*Delivery Dosages*	*Common Starting*
[Generic]	Minocycline	Capsule, tablet, liquid	50, 75, or 100 mg, twice a day
Minocin	Minocycline	Capsules, oral suspension	50 or 100 mg, twice a day
Dynacin	Minocycline	Capsules, tablets	50 or 100 mg, twice a day
Vectrin	Minocycline	Capsules	50, or 100 mg, twice a day

Minocycline is given in doses ranging from 50 milligrams twice a day to 100 milligrams once or twice a day. Minocycline's excellent absorption means it may be taken with food, even dairy products, without interfering with its efficacy, so you're less likely to get an upset stomach than if you were taking a "plain" tetracycline.

As with "plain" tetracycline and doxycycline, the dosage of the drug can be tapered when the inflammation has lessened.

Additional advantages of minocycline include

✔ Few, if any, sun-related problems.

✔ It appears to be less likely to induce vaginal yeast infections than plain tetracycline (see the section "Taking generic 'plain' tetracycline").

But, in addition to the expense, minocycline use includes other disadvantages:

✔ **Dizziness:** This side effect usually settles after a few days or when the dosage is lowered.

✔ **Skin pigmentation:** A reversible bluish darkening of the gums and/or skin may occur with long-term use.

✔ **Nausea:** Minocycline is more likely than plain tetracycline to cause such side effects as nausea, vomiting, and, in high doses (those that approach 200 milligrams per day), dizziness or vertigo.

✔ **Permanent tooth discoloration:** A very rare, irreversible blue discoloration of permanent teeth has been reported. Professional capping may be necessary to hide it.

One very rare, more serious side effect may exist with minocycline: A syndrome known as *drug-induced lupus erythematosus* occurs (most often in young women), and usually develops late in the course of therapy with minocycline. It has rarely proved fatal. The symptoms consist of swollen glands, rash, fever, and joint pains. This condition generally resolves within weeks or months of stopping minocycline.

Taking doxycycline

Doxycycline is also a tetracycline. It is available in generic formulations as well as brand names that I include in Table 10-3. In addition, doxycycline is available as a branded generic that goes by a number of names (see Chapter 9 for more on branded generics and Appendix B for a complete listing of brand-name acne drugs). It is somewhat less expensive and probably somewhat less effective than minocycline.

Table 10-3	The Doxycyclines		
Brand Name	**Generic Name**	**Delivery**	**Common Starting Dosages**
[Generic]	Doxycycline	Capsule, tablet, liquid	50, 75, or 100 mg, twice a day
Periostat	Doxycycline hyclate	Tablets	20 mg, twice a day
Adoxa	Doxycycline	Tablets	75 or 100 mg, twice a day

Doxycycline is given in doses ranging from 50 milligrams twice a day to 100 milligrams once or twice a day. It may also be prescribed to be taken as 75 milligrams once or twice a day. Doxycycline is well absorbed and may be taken with food. Taking it with food will make you less likely to get an upset stomach.

In addition to the slightly lower cost of doxycycline versus minocycline, another advantage of doxycycline is that the potential serious side effects sometimes seen with minocycline (dizziness, vertigo, skin darkening, and the lupus-like syndrome) have not been reported with doxycycline.

However, doxycycline's main disadvantage is its phototoxic potential — severe reactions to sun exposure— the highest of the tetracyclines. You should be advised about sun protection if you're prescribed this medication. Realistically, however, this is an uncommon side effect.

Low-dose doxycycline

Doxycycline, used in a very low dosage known as a *subantimicrobial* dose, is now being evaluated as a treatment for acne. Very low doses of doxycycline — as little as 20 milligrams twice a day — have been shown to have anti-inflammatory effects without acting upon *P. acnes*, the bacteria involved in producing acne. This approach is intended to avoid inducing bacterial resistance.

Studies on low-dose doxycycline have so far been done on people who have rosacea, a condition in which *P. acnes* doesn't seem to play any role, and some positive results have been noted on the inflammatory papules and pustules of rosacea that are very similar to those of acne (see Chapter 18). The question is whether it will also be effective in treating acne even if it doesn't suppress *P. acnes*.

Second-Line Oral Antibiotics

In some cases, tetracyclines may not work and your doctor will have to resort to some other oral antibiotic. Less commonly used oral antibiotics for moderate to severe inflammatory acne include

✔ **Erythromycin:** It's useful as a second-line alternative when tetracycline fails or isn't tolerated. Younger children (under age 10) can take it because it doesn't stain their teeth like tetracycline does. Although you should strive to avoid the use of oral drugs if you're pregnant, trying to become pregnant, or breastfeeding, in exceptional circumstances, erythromycin can be taken safely during these times. (See Chapter 5 for information on treating acne during pregnancy.)

There are a couple of drawbacks associated with erythromycin:

Bacterial resistance is a concern, and stomach upsets and diarrhea are not uncommon side effects of erythromycin. An *enterically coated* (designed to pass through the stomach undigested and into the intestines where they're absorbed) erythromycin product such as E-Mycin is less likely to cause gastrointestinal upsets and diarrhea.

As with the tetracyclines, erythromycin can permit vaginal yeast infections, known as *candidal vulvovaginitis,* to reappear. Candidal vulvovaginitis can also occur for the first time when taking erythromycin.

✔ **Amoxicillin:** This penicillin derivative is another safer alternative to a tetracycline that can be used during pregnancy.

✔ **Azithromycin (Zithromax):** The use of azithromycin, an antibiotic, as a four- or five-day pulse therapy in women who have monthly premenstrual acne flares has recently gained some interest. *Pulse therapy* (also called intermittent therapy) means not taking a medicine every day; rather it's taken, for example, for several days per week or for one week per month, discontinued, and then started again. The pattern repeats itself as necessary.

Other pulsing routines have been suggested to reduce the cost of this very expensive drug that is effective in the reduction of inflammatory acne lesions. Some dermatologists suggest that azithromycin is an alternative to tetracycline in patients with moderate to severe acne. It has no serious side effects; however, as with all of the antibiotics, buildup of bacterial resistance is a concern.

✔ **Clindamycin:** This antibiotic is a very effective acne fighter; however, the resistance pattern is similar to that of erythromycin and it has potentially serious side effects.

Furthermore, this drug has been associated with a severe type of gastrointestinal infection.

✔ **Cephalosporins:** The new-generation cephalosporin antibiotics appear to have good activity against acne. Again, bacterial resistance is a concern with these agents.

✔ **Trimethoprim sulfasoxazole (TMZ):** This is an oral sulfonamide that is very effective as an anti-acne agent. It is reserved for unusually stubborn cases of severe acne that don't respond to any of the other antibiotics listed here. It is sometimes used in situations in which Accutane (see Chapter 13) isn't appropriate.

TMZ has been associated with severe side effects and may precipitate severe allergic reactions. These reactions are quite rare. The development of resistance is also an issue.

Surveying Strategies to Reduce Antibiotic Use

I recommend that you make every effort to taper off oral antibiotics as soon as your acne is under control. An oral antibiotic may be intended for daily use over an extended period of time, often for four to six months and possibly much longer. Eventually, your doctor will taper off the medication and finally discontinue using it as your acne improves. The ideal long-term goal is to stop oral antibiotics altogether and rely only on topical therapy. In this section, I explain ways your doctor may decrease the total amount of antibiotic that you have to take while treating your acne.

If necessary, antibiotics may be continued at the lowest effective dose for long periods of time, especially if your acne is persistent. However, this practice can lead to antibiotic resistance. (See the "Addressing some common concerns" section, earlier in this chapter, to find out about bacterial resistance.)

But remember, always discuss these options with your doctor. Don't just change your doses on your own. Your doctor knows more about your skin and appropriate treatment for your acne than I do (unless of course you're one of my patients).

Rollercoastering is a term I use to describe a method of fine-tuning the dosage of oral antibiotics that may help to minimize some potential side effects, lessen the total dosage you take, and bring the cost of the medication down.

For example, a dosage schedule can begin with two 50 milligram minocycline capsules to be taken in the morning and one in the evening, which equals 150 milligrams per day. Because the highest recommended dosage is 200 milligrams in one day, this dosage allows for a possible increase of an additional 50 milligrams per day on your next follow-up visit to your dermatologist. However, if your acne shows marked improvement on the follow-up visit, your doctor may lower your dosage to say, 50 milligrams twice a day.

If you experience premenstrual flares of acne, talk to your doctor about increasing the dosage five to seven days before your next menstrual period and then lowering your dosage afterward.

Other ways to reduce the amount of antibiotics used to treat acne include pulsing (which I describe in the "Second-Line Oral Antibiotics" section, earlier in the chapter), using Accutane and other oral isotretinoins (see Chapter 13), and cortisone injections (see the sidebar in this chapter).

Your Guides to Your Medications

How did the doctor say that I should apply that cream? What were the side effects of that pill? Should I take it on an empty stomach or with food? If you're like most people, you probably don't remember half of what was said to you in your dermatologist's or healthcare provider's office.

Be sure to ask for written material about acne in general and also be sure you get written directions on how to use the medications that are prescribed for you. When you get home, make sure you read the material so that you understand the possible side effects, correct dosage, and everything else you need to know. If you have any questions, be sure to call your dermatologist or healthcare provider rather than waiting for your next office visit.

Your pharmacist should be a great resource for you. You can always ask for information about any of the drugs you were prescribed, as well as any of the over-the-counter drugs that you may be buying without a prescription. Better yet, ask your pharmacist for a printout that describes all of the actions and possible reactions you may experience with a prescription drug.

Getting needled: A possible substitute for antibiotics

A quick, relatively painless procedure, known as an intralesional cortisone (steroid) injection, is extremely effective in reducing the pain, swelling, and redness of acne papules or nodules (cysts). These shots are particularly effective for the larger, long-lasting lesions.

Each papule or nodule is given a single injection of a dilute cortisone solution, using a tiny, ultrathin needle.

The injection can hurt a little; however, within just a few days, the lesions soften, and in a week they become flat. Sometimes, the injections must be repeated in a month (or more) if the lesions aren't responding.

Many folks are needle-shy; however, after the first successful experience with this method, most come back asking for more. By the way, the bigger the cysts are, the less the needle hurts.

If too strong a concentration of cortisone is used, *atrophy,* or depressed scars that look like dents in the skin, may result at the injected sites. These dents usually resolve after several months, but they can be permanent. Similar atrophy may also have been the "normal" healing response of the inflamed lesion if it had not been injected.

The intralesional injections also serve as antibiotic sparers. If only a few lesions are present, say about one to five, these injections can serve as a substitute for oral antibiotics or allow your doctor to lower their dosages.

You can also turn to the *package insert* (the piece of paper that's supplied by the drug manufacturer), which has all that small print that describes every possible thing that has happened, or might happen, to anybody who takes the drug. It has more information than you'll ever need to know about the drug you were prescribed and it may convince you never to take it. See the "Looking at the package insert" sidebar in this chapter for more information.

If you desire, remember to ask your dermatologist or pharmacist whether there is a generic substitute for the prescribed medication. Check out Chapter 9 for more information on what generic medications are and how they can help you.

Looking at the package insert

Open up your package insert and check out the section named "adverse reactions" that lists all of the side effects that were reported in people and animals who were given the drug while it was being tested before going to market. These side effects can look frightening because they include so many problems, ranging from sneezing to life-threatening symptoms. The thing to remember is that this section lists *everything* that happened to thousands of people and/or animals during the testing phase regardless of whether it actually had any connection to the medicine.

It can be hard for you to decide which of the side effects on these lists you really need to be concerned about. You probably shouldn't be troubled about ones listed as rare or infrequent, unless they're also discussed in the "warnings" section. Even the side effects listed as being most frequent don't affect everyone who takes the medicine. Keep in mind, every person is different and it is impossible to tell in advance what you will experience.

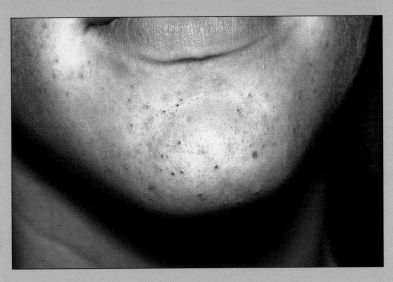

Acne vulgaris
This 14-year-old girl has blackheads (open comedones) on her chin. Also note the small red papules and macules on her chin.
See Chapter 4.

Acne vulgaris
This 16-year-old boy has small papules (A), a large pustule (B), and whiteheads — closed comedones (C).
See Chapter 4.

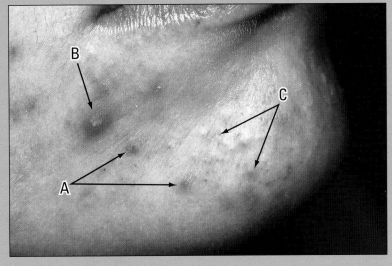

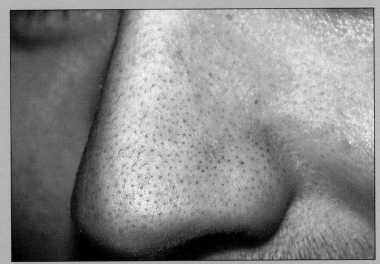

Follicular prominence
These little black holes look like blackheads, but they're actually open pores frequently seen on the nose and cheeks of people with acne.
See Chapter 9.

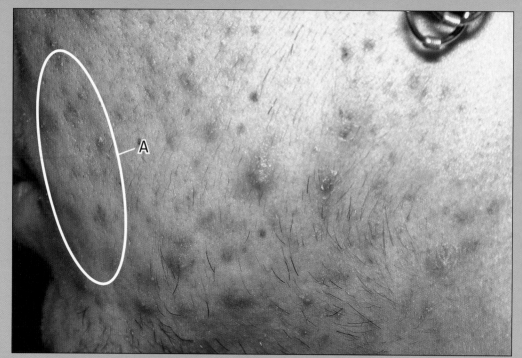

Acne vulgaris

This 17-year-old boy has severe inflammatory acne consisting of papules and pustules. There's also early evidence of pitted scarring (A). See Chapter 16.

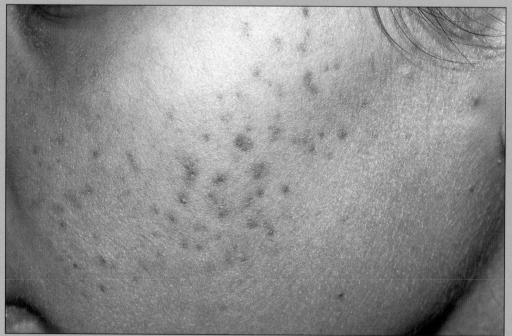

Courtesy of *Goodheart's Photoguide to Common Skin Disorders,* © Lippincotte Williams & Wilkins, 2003

Acne vulgaris

This young woman has small, flat, reddish-purple lesions — evidence of improvement from appropriate treatment (they were originally red papules). These blemishes heal slowly and most of them should disappear with further therapy. Some of them, however, may heal as "ice pick" scars. See Chapter 4.

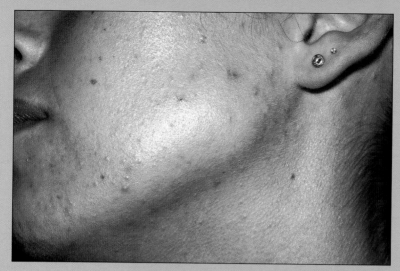

Adult-onset acne
The location of acne papules along the jaw line is characteristic of adult-onset acne in women. See Chapter 5.

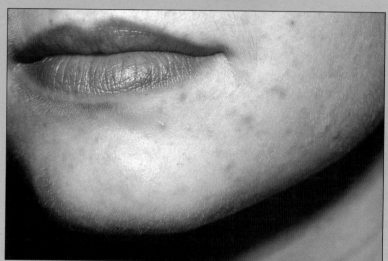

Adult-onset acne
These papules occurred like clockwork, right before this woman's period. See Chapter 5.

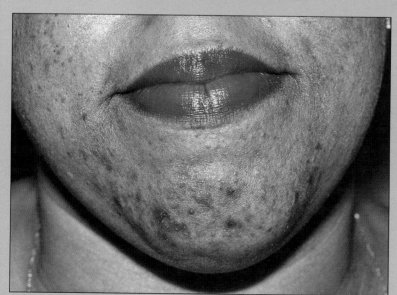

Adult-onset acne
Postinflammatory hyperpigmentation (PIP) is seen in this woman. When her acne lesions heal, they leave spots like the ones you can see on her chin. See Chapter 12.

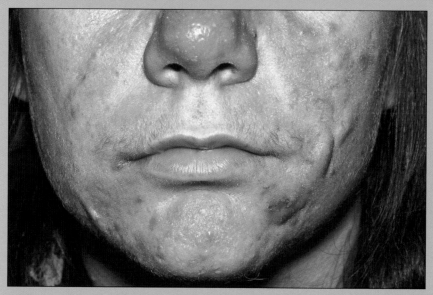

Severe nodular acne
This young woman had severe nodular acne that was unresponsive to all attempted treatments. See Chapter 13.

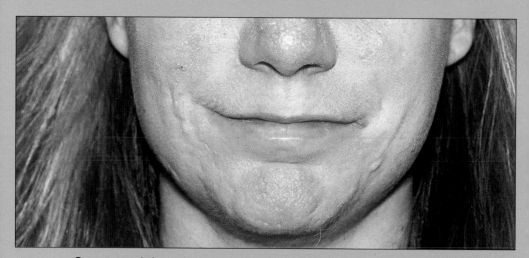

Severe nodular acne
This is the same woman after two 20-week courses of Accutane therapy. See Chapter 13.

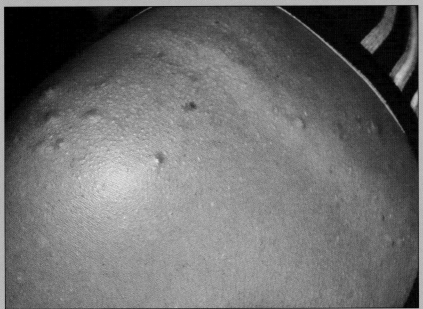

Hypertrophic scars

These scars, as seen on this young woman's shoulder, bulge out. They developed at the sites where the original inflammatory acne lesions healed. See Chapter 16.

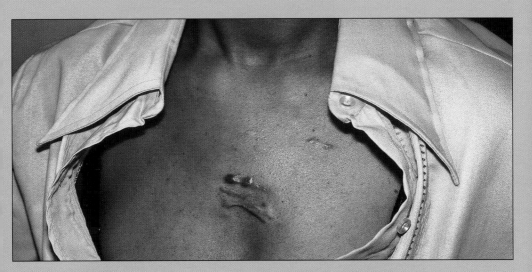

Keloids

These scars also arose from inflammatory lesions. The size of these scars goes beyond what would be expected from what was a minor acne lesion. See Chapter 16.

Rosacea

This 59-year-old woman has inflammatory papules, pustules, and broken blood vessels (telangiectasias) located on the central one-third of her face. See Chapter 18.

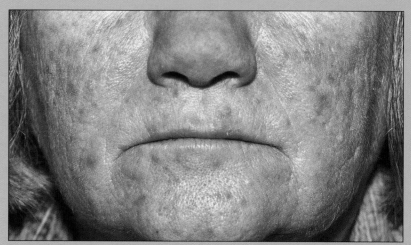

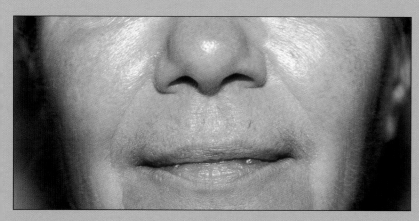

Rosy cheeks

This woman has rosy cheeks and telangiectasias. See Chapter 18.

Rosacea

This 64-year-old man has an enlarged nose with lumpy protuberances characteristic of rhinophyma. The excess tissue was later successfully removed with scalpel and laser surgery. See Chapter 18.

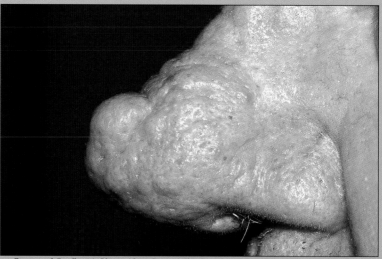

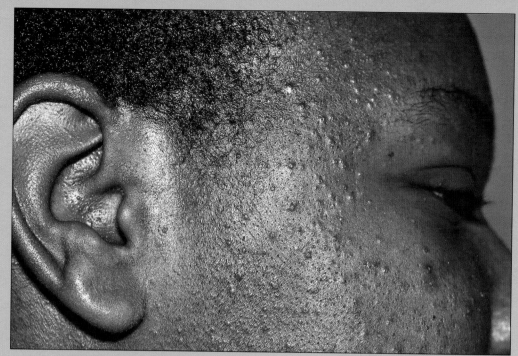

Pomade acne

This man has typical comedonal lesions due to hair greases and oils. Notice how they appear along his hairline and side of his face. See Chapter 12.

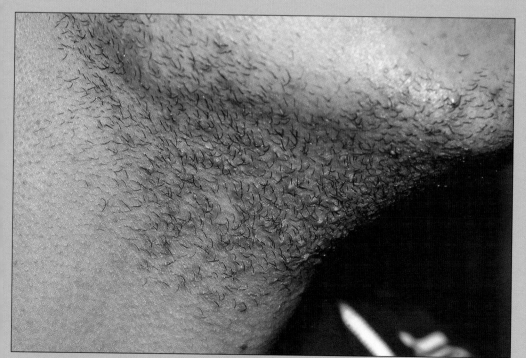

Razor bumps

This man has pseudofolliculitis barbae. Note the curved ingrowing hairs, papules, and pustules that resemble acne under the chin and on the upper neck. See Chapter 19.

Perioral dermatitis

This young woman has a ring of acne-like papules that circle her mouth, typical of the appearance of this condition. See Chapter 18.

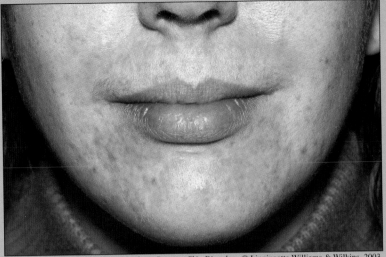

Courtesy of *Goodheart's Photoguide to Common Skin Disorders,* © Lippincotte Williams & Wilkins, 2003

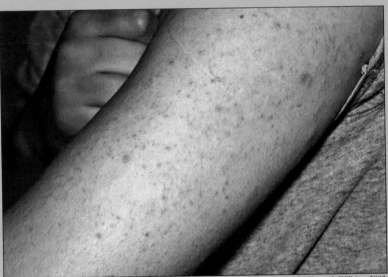

Keratosis pilaris

These are acne-like lesions seen on the upper-outer arm. If you were to rub your hand down this teenager's arms, they would feel rough-textured. See Chapter 19.

Courtesy of *Goodheart's Photoguide to Common Skin Disorders,* © Lippincotte Williams & Wilkins, 2003

Polycsystic ovary syndrome

Besides acne, this young woman has excess facial hair growth, diabetes, and menstrual irregularities. See Chapter 20.

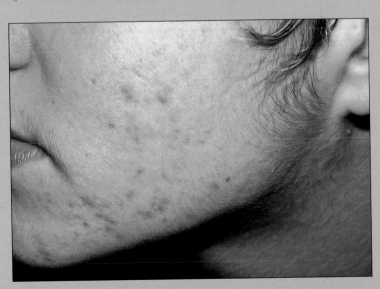

Chapter 11

Hormonal Treatment for Women

In This Chapter

▶ Deciding to use hormonal therapy

▶ Taking oral contraceptives to treat acne

▶ Figuring out if you have excessive androgens

▶ Adding anti-androgens to your regimen

*T*his chapter is for the females in the audience. Women often break out with acne in their 20s and early 30s, sometimes for the first time in their lives. This is thought to be hormone related and it is believed to be the main reason that more adult women than adult men have acne. And, of course, teenage girls, especially as they approach adulthood, also have the hormonal acne highs and lows that are generally less obvious than those seen in adult women.

Your *androgenic* or *male* hormones play a major role in the development of acne. (Yep, females have male hormones — just in smaller amounts than men do. For more on this topic, read Chapter 3.) As an adult, these male hormones can also encourage the onset and persistence of acne; in a nutshell, the androgens stimulate the sebaceous glands, enlarging them, and they produce excessive oil that promotes inflammatory acne. (For information on *how* androgens affect your skin, turn to Chapter 20.)

When the usual treatments such as topical measures and oral antibiotics that are listed in Chapters 9 and 10 aren't working well enough, the use of certain oral contraceptives can help to block the acne-causing response to your androgens. Many *oral contraceptives* (birth control pills) inhibit these androgens from stimulating your sebaceous glands to produce the oil that fuels your acne.

Hormonal therapy with an anti-androgen may be used in tandem with birth control pills when the pill alone isn't controlling acne or if you have, in addition to acne, some of the masculinizing symptoms of excess androgens such as excessive hair growth or thinning scalp hair.

Using Oral Contraceptives

When other measures fail to control your acne, you may want to consider birth control pills. The pill helps to level out the uneven surges of your estrogens and progesterone. Oral contraceptives may be a good choice for you if:

- ✔ You're sexually active and desire birth control pills
- ✔ You require oral hormonal therapy to regulate your menstrual cycle
- ✔ You're prescribed the drug Accutane (see Chapter 13)

Many women who have minimal to mild acne and who are also looking to use some form of contraception might discover that the pill alone can bring their acne under control. Moderate to severe acne can also be improved with a birth control pill that can be combined with topical and oral therapies.

If you're reluctant to take the pill or to use other birth control methods for moral or religious reasons, anti-androgens or physical treatments, such as laser or lights, are other therapeutic options that you and your doctor may consider. (I cover anti-androgens later in this chapter and lasers and lights in Chapter 14.)

Other means of hormonal birth control such as the birth control patch and ring have an unpredictable effect on acne and can actually provoke it at times. Depo-Provera, an injection containing synthetic progesterone, can also worsen or trigger acne at times (see the section "Suppressing the cycle — and the acne," later in this chapter).

There are both negative and positive side effects to taking birth control pills for acne. Talk to your doctor to decide if it is right for you.

Birth control pills are often prescribed to prevent pregnancy in females who are given isotretinoin (Accutane), unless they've had a hysterectomy or are otherwise physically incapable of getting pregnant. Accutane is a powerful drug for treating severe acne that has been associated with severe birth defects. Besides abstinence, birth control pills are considered to be the preferred method of contraception for women who are taking Accutane. I talk about Accutane in Chapter 13.

Suppressing the cycle — and the acne

Oral contraceptives have been available since the 1960s. They prevent ovulation and make conditions difficult for a fertilized egg to implant on the uterus wall.

The goal of oral contraceptives in treating your acne is to block the effects of your androgens on your sebaceous glands. Oral contraceptives contain estrogen, which regulates menstruation. Besides suppressing ovulation, the estrogens in birth control pills can help improve acne by:

- ✔ Reducing ovarian androgen secretion
- ✔ Blocking the androgens that are produced from stimulating your sebaceous glands to produce excess oil (they act as *androgen receptor blockers* in medspeak)

The estrogens have the ability to decrease the levels of your *free testosterone* (androgen). They do this by increasing the amount of *sex hormone binding globulin* (SHBG), a protein that "mops up" your free testosterone, hangs onto it, and doesn't allow it to stimulate your acne-producing oil glands to produce excess oil.

Oral contraceptives that are most helpful in controlling acne are those that contain a combination of an estrogen and a *progestin* (synthetic progesterone).

The *minipill,* the progestin-only pill, is an effective oral contraceptive with fewer side effects than the combination pill. However, its effects on acne are unpredictable. Progestins have effects that can be *androgenic* (acting like male hormones). Some of the newer progestins have less androgenic activity and therefore are less likely to worsen, and may improve, your acne.

If you're over 35 years of age, have migraine headaches, or are a cigarette smoker, birth control pills that contain estrogen are not for you!

Taking the best pills for acne

Taking oral contraceptives may improve your acne even if you have no evidence of excess androgen production. In fact, the level of testosterone in most women who have acne is within the normal range, but the levels can be lowered and blocked if you're taking the right pill.

Most dermatologists recommend use of the *low-dose oral contraceptives*, which are oral contraceptive combinations with minimal androgenicity. These drugs increase SHBG and thus decrease androgen concentrations in healthy women.

The oral contraceptives Ortho Tri-Cyclen, Estrostep, and Yasmin are the best ones to take if you have acne. Yasmin, in addition to an estrogen, has as its progestin, *drospirenone,* which is a very close chemical relative to *spironolactone,* a very potent antiandrogenic hormone that is described in the next section. Many dermatologists feel that Yasmin is the most effective oral contraceptive available for the treatment of acne.

Several of these oral contraceptives are packaged in convenient dosing schedules and come in packets of 28 tablets. The first 21 tablets are the active pills; they contain the *active ingredients,* hormones. (I explain what active ingredients are in Chapter 7.) The last 7 tablets in a 28-tablet packet are the reminder pills (that contain inactive ingredients); they're different in color and don't contain any hormone.

Read the package label and follow directions as indicated.

Other oral contraceptives that have low androgenicity include Levlen, Levlite, Seasonale, Tri-Levlen, Triphasil, Desogen, and Alesse.

Diane-35, is approved in Canada, and has been approved for two decades in Europe as an oral contraceptive that is very effective in the treatment of acne, but it isn't available in the United States. It contains *cyproterone*, an androgen receptor blocker and potent progestin.

Be patient. It may take at least three months on the pill before you see positive results for your acne.

Looking out for side effects

Although the original oral contraceptives had a number of side effects, they've been modified to reduce their risks. Historically, the most serious side effect of birth control pills had been that of *thromboembolism* (blood clots) that begin in the veins of the legs. However, the present lower doses of estrogens have all but eliminated this potential complication.

Other potential side effects include:

- ✔ **Nausea, vomiting, abdominal cramping, or bloating:** These problems are the most common minor side effects. They usually go away as the body adjusts to the drug.

- ✔ **Headaches:** These tend to be mild, but if they become severe, discuss the problem with your doctor.

- ✔ **Spotting and breakthrough bleeding:** Irregular vaginal bleeding or spotting may occur while you are taking the pills.

- ✔ **Slight weight gain:** This may occur due to an increase in your appetite.

- ✔ **Mood swings (depression, anxiety):** The hormonal disruption caused by the pill may result in mood swings and a lowering of libido.

- ✔ **Breast tenderness:** Swollen, tender breasts and/or breast lumps that are not cancerous can occur.

Tell your doctor if you have or have ever had problems with your breasts such as lumps, an abnormal mammogram (breast X-ray), or fibrocystic breast disease. But most studies suggest that pills neither reduce nor increase the risk for breast cancer. Early detection is the key to successful breast cancer treatment and survival. Doing breast self-exams is easy, and the more you do it, the better you'll get at it. Better yet, mammography, particularly those using the latest MRI equipment, will find small tumors before you are able to feel them.

If you're taking the pill, you need to be counseled about its risks and you should have regular Pap smears and breast exams. A Pap smear is a test that checks the cells on the cervix (the opening of the uterus) for changes, which could lead to cancer.

Combination birth control pills (those that combine an estrogen and a progestin) apparently *lower* the risk of uterine and ovarian cancer according to recent studies.

Antibiotics and the pill

For a long time, it was assumed that there was an increase in the failure rate of birth control pills when women also took commonly used antibiotics such as the tetracyclines and erythromycins at the same time they were on the pill. A recent study has concluded that these antibiotics that are regularly used to treat acne probably *don't* interfere with the efficacy of oral contraceptives. Basically, if you're taking a tetracycline or an erythromycin antibiotic for your acne, you should be aware of this controversy so that you can decide if you wish to use an alternative or additional form of birth control. Many pharmacists are still giving patients this warning, largely because many birth control pill package inserts still contain this information.

The effect of oral contraceptives is unpredictable, everybody is different, and you may have to try several different ones before finding the right one that works on *your* acne.

Trying Anti-androgens

Instead of the typical anti-acne drugs and birth control pills, you may need specific anti-androgen treatment to control your acne. Anti-androgen treatment is an option when conventional topical and systemic therapies aren't working, you can't or don't wish to take a birth control pill, or when an endocrine abnormality is found in which your body is producing too many androgens.

Most healthcare providers recommend that you continue taking an oral contraceptive while taking most anti-androgens, because there is a risk of feminization of a male fetus if you become pregnant while taking either one of them. Ask your doctor for further details.

If you've noticed that some of your acne medications that previously worked have stopped being effective — the oral antibiotics, topical medications, and even birth control pills are no longer performing — you've had a relapse after taking a course of Accutane, or your acne has suddenly become severe, your doctor will likely evaluate you for *androgen excess.* Check out Chapter 20 where I discuss this condition and other endocrine disorders.

Spironolactone is the antiandrogen most frequently used to treat acne. An oral antiandrogen such as spironolactone (Aldactone) is used in women in whom hormonal treatment may be an effective alternative, or as an accompaniment to oral contraceptives and antibiotics. It is useful for women with recurrent outbreaks of deep inflammatory nodules. Spironolactone has potent antiandrogenic effects, and it works by decreasing sebum production.

Spironolactone is started at a low dosage of 25 to 50 milligrams per day and may be increased. It may take three months to notice any positive effects, but results may appear sooner. The dosage may need to be adjusted during the first six months of treatment.

Your dermatologist or healthcare provider may order certain blood tests while you're taking this medication.

The most common side effect of this drug is an irregular menstrual cycle; however, if you're taking birth control pills, this is less likely to happen. Breast tenderness sometimes occurs. Women with a personal history, or strong family history, of breast cancer should discuss the risks and benefits of taking this drug with their doctor. But after more than 50 years of using this drug in humans, there is no evidence — except in mice — that it causes any kind of cancer.

Spironolactone is sometimes used to treat *hypertension* (high blood pressure) as a *diuretic* (water pill). If you're already taking a medication for high blood pressure such as a diuretic, you might ask your doctor to substitute spironolactone for one of the water pills or other blood pressure drugs you're taking. This approach might help treat your acne and high blood pressure at the same time.

Flutamide (Eulexin) is another anti-androgen that is sometimes used in unmanageable female adult acne. It has the potential of causing severe liver damage, which greatly limits its use.

A minimum of three to six months of therapy is required for you and your healthcare provider to evaluate the efficacy of these antiandrogen agents.

Chapter 12

Managing Acne in Dark-Complexioned Skin

*A*cne is an equal-opportunity skin disorder. It occurs in people of all races and ethnicities. It has the same causes and follows a similar course in people with all shades of skin. However, there are some differences in the appearance and treatment of acne among different groups. This chapter covers the methods to prevent and treat these distinctive issues as well as suggesting approaches for skin-care in darker skin populations.

Recognizing Diversity

Variations among skin tones all come down to *melanin,* which is responsible for absorbing sunlight and giving your skin its distinctive color. As I explain in Chapter 2, melanin is produced in *melanocytes* (pigment-producing cells). Everyone has the same number of melanocytes; however, in more darkly pigmented people, these pigment-producing factories create more melanin and are inclined to disperse it more widely in the epidermis.

There are important medical and cosmetic advantages to having dark skin. Darker skin is more resistant to sunburns, skin cancer, and wrinkles. As dark skin ages, the higher melanin content and facial oil cause the skin to age less rapidly than lighter skin.

However, dark skin does have disadvantages when it comes to dealing with acne — dark spots and scars are more likely to appear (more about that later in the chapter).

Our world is host to great variability in skin color among people of all races. We're all pretty much the same underneath where it counts, and making generalizations about acne and race or skin color is difficult.

But, the following are some of the features that are more likely to be seen in darker skin types:

- ✔ Dark spots are often the number one concern to the person with acne. Check out the next section that talks about how they form and what you can do about them.

- ✔ Inflammatory (red) acne lesions tend to be less visible. Lesions *appear* to be less common in very dark skin because the red color of inflammation is often well hidden by the surrounding darker skin.

- ✔ Sensitive skin known as *eczema* (atopic dermatitis) is more common in Asians, African-Americans, and Hispanics.

- ✔ Healing acne lesions tend to produce larger scars in Hispanics, Asians, and particularly African-Americans, as compared to Caucasians. (I discuss scars in Chapter 16.)

The good news is that people of color are less likely to have severe nodular acne than are Caucasians.

Figuring Out Those Dark Spots!

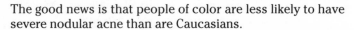

People with white skin tend to complain about red marks that remain red or purplish in color. These spots are called *macules* in dermatologese. Like freckles and tattoos, they're simply color changes of the skin (you can't feel macules, and if you close your eyes, they don't exist).

In black skin, those same red spots look much darker, even deep brown or black in color and many shades in between, particularly after they heal. African-Americans are often more concerned about these dark acne-related macules than they are about the acne itself. The dark spots are known as *postinflammatory hyperpigmentation* or *postinflammatory pigmentation* — or PIP for short. To see what PIP looks like, turn to the color section of this book.

How dark spots are formed

PIP is limited to the sites of previous inflammation. Think of the spots as "footprints," the aftermath or telltale signs that show where the original injury (inflammatory "battle") took place. The original insult (and injury) that caused PIP can be a cut, a burn, a rash, or the after-effect from a healing acne lesion.

Often these "footprints" disappear over a period of time, but they always outlast the original inflammatory acne lesions themselves. In fact, they may take many months or even years to fade completely.

There are actually two types of PIP. Both start off when inflammation of the skin, such as acne, stimulates the melanocytes in your epidermis and causes them to step up the manufacturing of melanin. The production of melanin *(melanogenesis)* increases in response to the tanning effect of sun, injuries to the skin such as burns, cuts, surgeries, as well as the inflammation caused by acne.

The two different types of PIP are

- ✔ **Epidermal hypermelanosis:** The busy melanocytes respond by handing off their melanin pigment in tiny granules to surrounding *keratinocytes,* your other epidermal cells. This increased stimulation and transfer of melanin granules results in *epidermal hypermelanosis.* Your skin gets darker, but the pigment isn't deep.

  The good news is that this type of PIP often responds to topical bleaching creams, which help to accelerate its disappearance. That's because the majority of the melanin pigment is in the epidermis (the top layer of the skin) which allows it to be treated.

- ✔ **Dermal melanosis:** *Dermal melanosis* occurs when inflammation disrupts the basal cell layer, causing melanin pigment to be released and subsequently "dropped" more deeply into the dermis where it gets trapped by *macrophages* (scavenger white cells). This type of PIP is much harder to treat and may never fade away completely.

These spots are *not* scars, and some, if not all, of them will fade in time, or if necessary, they can be lightened with appropriate treatment (see tips for treating them later in this section). Unless the pigment is very deep, PIP will improve over time. Be an extra patient patient! The dark spots take the longest to fade. The treatment of PIP tends to be a difficult and prolonged process that often takes 6 to 12 months to achieve the desired results of depigmentation.

Preventing PIP

Keisha is a 30-year-old woman who started developing acne in her late 20s. When I first saw her, the first words out of her mouth were, "What can you do to help get rid of these scars?" She was referring to dark spots on her cheeks and forehead. "They won't go away. I hate them," she said.

I looked closely at her skin and told her that she didn't have scars. Those dark spots were where her acne had healed; the spots were PIP. I examined her more thoroughly and noted that she did have active acne lesions on her face in addition to the "inactive" dark spots.

I explained to her that her "active" acne lesions caused those spots and that our first priority was to treat and prevent the "hot spots" and let the dark spots take care of themselves.

We began by treating her acne, and when she returned six weeks later, her acne was getting under control and the dark spots were beginning to fade. After a total of three months of treatment, her skin tone was evening out and she was quite pleased.

I reassured her that if any of the dark spots remained after six to eight months of the current treatment, I would give her additional medications to apply to try to bleach them.

Deterring the dark spots

Because these spots can take so long to disappear, it's essential to prevent them from appearing in the first place. Early treatment and prevention of your acne can help put a stop to them. You should be aware of those things that put you at greater risk of developing PIP. For example, you should avoid:

- ✔ Squeezing, rubbing, or picking your acne lesions

- ✔ Over-the-counter toners, witch hazel, and alcohol products as well as prescription acne products that may dry and irritate your skin and lead to PIP

- ✔ Harsh soaps and overwashing (for tips on how to properly wash your face, see Chapter 2)

- ✔ Scrubbing with loofahs and buff puffs

- ✔ Cosmetics that might aggravate your skin and make your acne look worse

I know, it's tempting to think that squeezing spots will help them heal more quickly. In fact, squeezing actually makes them worse. Squeezing a spot carries a risk of scarring because the pus can burst inward *into* the skin rather than *outward* to the surface.

In fact, any situation where the skin can be irritated, be it squeezing blemishes, or plucking hair, can result in dark skin's tendency to produce more melanin and create dark spots.

Shaving the beard can also wreak havoc with acne and increase the possibility to develop PIP. Check out Chapter 19, where I provide some helpful tips on gentle shaving techniques.

Keeping Acne and Dark Spots at Bay with OTC Medications

The same medications that are used to treat acne in Caucasian skin are also used to treat people of color; however, when there is a potential to develop PIP, you sometimes need to use the medications differently.

If after eight weeks of self-treatment, your acne and your dark spots persist, seek professional help from your healthcare provider or a dermatologist. In Chapter 8, I tell you how to find the right professional to help you treat your acne.

PIP may further darken with sun exposure, so to be truly effective, any therapy should include applying a sunblock over any acne or bleaching medications you use. Other measures to limit ultraviolet exposure (for example wearing hats, protective clothing, and — the best option — avoiding the sun altogether) should be part of your routine.

Benzoyl peroxide and salicylic acid

Over-the-counter (or OTC) medications such as benzoyl peroxide and salicylic acid may be an excellent approach if your acne is mild and you're able to tolerate these products, but they can be quite irritating on some people's skin. I discuss these products in greater detail in Chapter 7.

Begin with a benzoyl peroxide preparation. If your skin is able to tolerate it and you see improvement of your acne, stick with it. If you want a further boost to your treatment, try adding an over-the-counter salicylic acid at another time of day or just apply it over the benzoyl peroxide.

Apply a sunscreen over any medication(s) you are using.

Benzoyl peroxide and salicylic acid can be irritating and drying and produce whitish scales on dark skin. These scales are often referred to as looking "ashy." The appearance of the scales is difficult for some people to tolerate. (Light skin or white skin gets ashy too; it's just that you don't see the contrast as well.)

If benzoyl peroxide or salicylic acid is producing ashiness and scales, apply a light non-oily moisturizer like Cetaphil Moisturizing Cream or Olay Active Hydrating Beauty Fluid. If you have dark spots, use a moisturizer that contains a sunscreen such as Purpose Moisturizer SPF 15 or Cetaphil Daily Facial Moisturizer SPF 15. If you prefer, you may use a heavier, greasier moisturizer.

If you have sensitive skin, be sure to use the lower strength (like 2.5 percent benzoyl peroxide water-based) products to start with. Start treatment every second night, then build up to once or twice daily, as you're able to tolerate the product. Similarly, if you get too ashy or irritated from salicylic acid products that have a mild peeling activity, try using the lower 1 percent concentration or try applying the medications on an alternate-day basis.

Over-the-counter bleaches

For the PIP spots, look for over-the-counter preparations that contain 1 to 2 percent hydroquinone, a chemical that's traditionally been the main treatment for PIP. Companies that make over-the-counter hydroquinone-containing "fade" creams and gels include Ambi, Esoterica, Porcelana, and Black Opal. These products are applied as a thin layer on the affected areas once or twice a day.

You may experience a mild skin irritation or temporary skin darkening. If skin irritation or darkening persists, stop using them and seek professional help.

If no improvement is seen after three months of treatment, their application should be discontinued.

Some of these agents contain a built-in sunscreen, however, sun exposure should be limited further by using an additional sun-blocking agent or protective headgear to shade treated skin or lightened skin.

The over-the-counter products may be helpful, but if they aren't strong enough, you may require one of the prescription strength medications that I describe later in this chapter.

There are over-the-counter products containing 10 percent hydroquinone or higher that are available in many other countries, particularly within Africa and Asia, and some of them have found their way (illegally) into "health" stores in the United States — mostly in ethnic neighborhoods within big cities. These high concentrations actually bring the risk of a *darkening reaction* known as *ochronosis.*

Getting Professional Help

Acne treatments are generally as safe and effective on dark skin as they are on light skin. And in most cases, the treatments are the same. In Chapters 8 through 11, I outline the topical and oral approaches that dermatologists commonly suggest and that are also appropriate for people with darker skin. The main difference in the professional treatment of darker skin is a deeper concern for skin discoloration or scars from acne.

In this section, I fill you in on how treatments differ when used on darker skin, including aggressive treatments of the acne and the use of more potent skin lighteners for PIP. When treating dark skin, a combination of topical creams and gels, chemical peels (see the "Treating your acne and PIP with topical drugs" section, later in the chapter), and sunscreens may be necessary for significant improvement. This combination of various topical therapeutic agents has been shown to be beneficial, especially on the face.

Daily use of a broad-spectrum sunscreen (SPF 15 or greater) is an essential part of any therapeutic regimen. This step is very important to prevent the pigmentation from becoming darker or allowing the already lightened skin to repigment.

The treatment of PIP tends to be a difficult and prolonged process and may not work at all. When it does work, it often takes 6 to 12 months to achieve cosmetically acceptable depigmentation.

Treating your acne and PIP with topical drugs

A variety of topical treatments have been used to treat epidermal PIP, with varying degrees of success. These agents include chemical peels, retinoids, azelaic acid, and hydroquinone. Lightening of dark areas may be achieved with one of these topical measures.

Each of these treatment options potentially improves epidermal hypermelanosis, but none are proven effective with dermal hypermelanosis.

Bleaching with prescription-strength hydroquinone

Hydroquinone is the cornerstone agent in the treatment of PIP. It's a topical bleaching agent that suppresses the melanocytes from producing melanin. Hydroquinone-containing combination products such as EpiQuin Micro, Glyquin XM, Lustra-AF, and Triluma are available by prescription only. Some of these agents contain their own sunscreens. In addition, some contain vitamin E, vitamin C, retinol, or glycolic acid.

There are unsubstantiated claims that some of these chemicals have "age-defying," sun-blocking, wrinkle-preventing properties when mixed with the hydroquinone. I really can't give you any opinion on those claims because with such a mixture of ingredients, it's hard to tell what each one does.

Hydroquinone may be prescribed along with azelaic acid (described later in the next section) to lighten the dark areas more quickly.

Preparations that contain hydroquinone are applied twice a day to the dark spots. Allergic reactions to them are rare.

Hydroquinone combination products are very expensive and are almost never covered by prescription plans because hyperpigmentation is considered a "cosmetic problem" for which treatment is "not medically necessary." I tell you this so you don't suffer "sticker shock" when you go to the pharmacy.

Some dermatologists will ask that a more concentrated prescription (up to 8 percent hydroquinone, instead of the usual 3 to 4 percent) be mixed (compounded) for you if you don't respond to the lower strength treatments.

Applying azelaic acid

Some products actually treat acne *and* bleach PIP, saving you money and valuable application time. *Azelaic acid,* a prescription product known as Azelex or Finerin, is an inhibitor of melanin synthesis. It can treat your acne and lighten the dark spots at the same time. Apply a small amount once or twice a day to all acne-prone areas including the dark spots. For more information on azelaic acid, see Chapter 9. Acne tends to respond to azelaic acid in six to eight weeks; however, the PIP spots may take many months to lighten.

Because azelaic acid decreases pigmentation, it can temporarily lighten areas that aren't targets of your treatment. It can also be irritating.

Relying on retinoids

Topical retinoids can also perform a double duty. In addition to the beneficial actions of the retinoids in treating and preventing both comedonal and inflammatory acne, they also may have a lightening effect on PIP. Adaplene (Differin), tazarotene (Tazorac), Avita, and tretinoin (Retin-A) are all prescription retinoids. See Chapter 9 for a complete discussion of these medications.

Retinoids are known to *hasten the rate of turnover* (get rid of dead cells, in plain English) of epidermal *keratinocytes* (the majority of the cells that make up the epidermis) and they also seem to assist in the normalization of pigmentation as well. Furthermore, by causing the skin to peel, they enhance the penetration of the other bleaching medications into the epidermis.

Creams are the least irritating, so you probably should start out with a cream-based retinoid instead of a gel. If you have oily skin or have a low risk for irritation, you may be prescribed a gel formulation with a higher concentration of retinoid in it.

Topical retinoids can be effective; however, they can be a "double-edged sword" if you have very sensitive skin. These products may result in more irritation that may ultimately cause more PIP.

Peeling the pigment away

It's possible to actually remove some layers of skin over time to remove layers of the pigment. The following procedures should be approached with great caution and performed only by a professional with a lot of experience in their use (for more details on these procedures, check out Chapter 14). The risk of worsening the PIP is always present with all of these procedures.

Chemical peels

Glycolic or salicylic acid peels can be effective treatments of PIP in dark-complexioned individuals. These are superficial peels that don't penetrate below the upper layers of skin, and they can sometimes help to even irregular skin tones and lighten PIP. Matching the strength of a peel to an individual's skin type and scarring history is critical to avoiding complications.

Salicylic and glycolic acids may be applied by an experienced dermatologist or cosmetic surgeon. They may need to perform the peel multiple times in order to see improvement. Depending on the strength of the acid peel, you may be asked to discontinue applying some or all of the topical agents that are described in the previous sections for a few days before the peel, and resume using them several weeks after the peel, to maintain the results.

These procedures need to be approached cautiously as the risk of peel-induced PIP is well known, as well as the risk of hypertrophic scarring and keloid formation that tends to occur to the more darkly complexioned individual. In Chapter 16, I tell you more about hypertrophic scars and keloids.

Lasers

Certain lasers are now being used to treat PIP, but should only be used by experienced medical professionals. People with dark skin have been told in the past that laser treatments aren't safe for them. But experts using the lower powered treatments at very specific wavelengths that are now available can help you avoid complications, such as exacerbating PIP or producing scars.

Microdermabrasion

This procedure is a superficial exfoliation that may not be suitable for skin of color, but it is sometimes used to treat PIP and smooth skin texture. It can be effective in reducing superficial hyperpigmentation; however, pigmentary streaking and worsening of PIP may occur in people with dark skin types.

Managing the scars

Acne scars can form after cysts and nodules heal. Even minor outbreaks of inflammatory acne can result in significant scarring if you're predisposed to form larger scars as is the case in many African-Americans.

Acne scars are difficult to treat, and *keloids,* large scars that grow way beyond the bounds of normal scars, are particularly difficult to deal with. *Intralesional cortisone injections,* though, are particularly effective for patients of color. As with inflammatory nodules and cysts, cortisone injections are sometimes injected directly into the scars to help shrink them. In these instances, higher concentrations than are used to treat active acne lesions are used. Other procedures, such as soft tissue fillers, scar revision, and laser surgery, may also be considered (see Chapter 16).

Caution must be used with all of these procedures because of the risk of creating further scarring and PIP. Therefore, only an experienced dermatologist or other cosmetic surgeon who is knowledgeable about skin of color should perform these corrective procedures. The method known as *dermabrasion,* used to remove deep scars, can sometimes be too risky to use on people with dark skin because it has a likelihood that it will make scarring and PIP worse.

The newest treatment of keloids and hypertrophic scars is to have them shaved flat or *excised* (cut out) by a dermatologist or plastic surgeon. After the procedure is done, the patient applies topical imiquimod (Aldara) cream for at least 8 weeks. There have been optimistic reports that there are fewer recurrences with this method.

Oral acne therapy to prevent scars and PIP

The use of oral therapy doesn't differ much according to the relative lightness or darkness of one's skin. But sometimes a more aggressive approach with oral antibiotics such as one of the oral tetracyclines (see Chapter 10) will get the less visible, "under-the-skin" papules and nodules under control and prevent the more obvious postinflammatory hyperpigmentation (PIP) and the more complicated hypertrophic scars and keloids that can result from them. Scar treatment is covered in Chapter 16.

Looking at Pomade Acne

African-Americans and other individuals who have tight curly hair frequently use *pomades* (oils and greasy ointments) to style or improve their hair's manageability. Some people believe that pomade acne is caused by the pomade's blockage of pores and that as a result, many pomade users develop blackheads and whiteheads, with perhaps a few papules and pustules on the forehead and/or temples — places where the pomade comes into contact with their skin. To see what pomade acne looks like, take a look at the color section of the book.

Pomades can also contribute to an inflammation or infection of the scalp, called *folliculitis,* in which pustules and redness develop around the hairs. This type of folliculitis can cause hair loss and scarring of the scalp. I talk about hair follicle problems in Chapter 19.

My best advice to you is to stop using pomades. If your acne persists after stopping, be sure to see a dermatologist. However, if you feel your life or hairstyle can't be complete without pomade, you still have a couple options to reduce potential problems:

- ✔ If you're using pomade to deal with a dry scalp, try applying the pomade 1 inch behind your hairline.

- ✔ If you're using it to style or make your hair more manageable, try applying the pomade to the ends of your hair only, to avoid contact with your scalp and hairline.

Cosmetics for Women of Various Ethnic Groups

Dark-complexioned women tend to be more concerned about skin tone and having a clear, even complexion than they are about wrinkles and fine lines.

Until recently, most skin-care companies have neglected African-Americans and other ethnic consumers. Ethnic cosmetic brands were available, but their products were far fewer than those in Caucasian makeup lines.

In the past decade, things have markedly improved and there are now many companies that offer skin-care products for women of color. The color spectrum has broadened to include a wider variety of darker color shades for you to match your skin tones and conceal your acne while not irritating or worsening it. Products for Asian women are still few in number; however, Shiseido now offers a full line of products for the Asian woman. Your dermatologist may be able to recommend cosmetic measures to make the PIP spots less apparent until they resolve.

You may have a problem in choosing the right cosmetic if you have uneven skin tones that represent an uneven distribution of your pigmentation, such as appears in PIP. Some areas are darker while some appear lighter. In such cases, you should match your foundation to the most predominant color, or find one with a shade in between the two. Experiment and sample before you buy. Pigmented makeup creams have also been successfully used to camouflage hyperpigmented skin to a shade similar to that of the surrounding unaffected skin.

Some companies can custom-blend foundation colors, but this may be very expensive; Dermablend (www.dermablend.com) and Covermark (www.covermark.com) are two such products. They're available in many shades that can be easily blended to match any skin tone. In fact, they can be used for people of all skin colors. Besides acne spots, they can be used to conceal skin imperfections such as birthmarks, burns, and discolorations from surgery. These products can be found in makeup counters in some department stores and also can be obtained online.

Of course, PIP occurs just as often in males; however, most males would not use camouflaging methods as readily as females to try to hide it.

Chapter 13

Attacking Acne with Accutane and Other Isotretinoins

● ●

In This Chapter

▶ Going over the terminology

▶ Getting to know isotretinoin

▶ Preparing for treatment

▶ Taking your medicine

● ●

*I*f your acne is really severe and hasn't responded to other types of therapy, your dermatologist may turn to *isotretinoin,* commonly known by its original brand name, Accutane. Isotretinoin is a powerful oral medication and, so far, it's the only treatment that induces a long-term, drug-free remission of severe acne.

The vast majority of people who have taken isotretinoin bear witness to the dramatic reduction in acne symptoms and a prolonged improvement they've experienced even after only one course of 15 to 20 weeks of isotretinoin. Okay, then, why don't I and all the other dermatologists out there simply install an isotretinoin vending machine in our waiting room?

There are three main reasons why isotretinoin treatment must be closely monitored (I thoroughly cover all three in this chapter):

✔ If taken during pregnancy, isotretinoin is highly likely to cause severe birth defects.

✔ There are many other possible side effects that can occur with isotretinoin use. They range in seriousness from dry lips to persistent headaches and temporary hearing loss.

> ✔ Isotretinoin may be linked to an increased risk of depression and suicide in people who take it.

Before going any further, I must tell you that most dermatologists believe that for those who have severe acne, the benefits of isotretinoin far outweigh the risks if the drug is taken as prescribed and specific cautions are followed. In this chapter, I explain why we're of this opinion and I give you details about the drug and precautions you can — and must — take, including the new program established in the United States to regulate access to this drug. But, as only your doctor can prescribe isotretinoin, he has the definitive word on all aspects of your treatment, so follow instructions and ask questions. And for before and after photos of a woman who has taken isotretinoin, see the color section of this book.

You Say Accutane, I Say Isotretinoin

Isotretinoin (its chemical name is *13-cis-retinoic acid*) is related to both tretinoin (retinoic acid) and retinol (vitamin A). Isotretinoin is derived from vitamin A, which makes it a *retinoid*. (I discuss topical retinoids that dermatologists prescribe in Chapter 9.) In Canada, the United Kingdom, Australia, and Europe, isotretinoin is available as a topical, as well as an oral, preparation to treat acne.

When isotretinoin is taken orally, it's classified as a *teratogen,* which means that it's a substance that can cause deformities in a fetus.

The original brand names for oral isotretinoin were Accutane in the United States and Roaccutane in rest of the world. Besides, Accutane and Roaccutane, it's now sold under several generic brand names in the United States, including

> ✔ Amnesteem
>
> ✔ Claravis
>
> ✔ Sotret

For our purposes, I simplify matters and simply call it isotretinoin. (For a complete listing of isotretinoin brand names in your neck of the woods, check out my guide to acne drugs around the world in Appendix B.)

Getting to Know the Drug and Its Uses

Isotretinoin is so effective because it has the ability to hit specific targets at the root of acne. (In Chapter 3, I go into all of the details about how acne forms.) Isotretinoin treats acne by:

- ✔ **Stopping the excess oil production:** Isotretinoin dramatically reduces the size and output of your sebaceous glands. It limits the amount of sebum and thus cuts off the acne bacteria's (technically known as *P. acnes*) food supply. Stemming the flow of oil explains the many drying side effects that I describe later in this chapter.

- ✔ **Stabilizing keratinization:** *Keratinization* is the process through which *keratinocytes* (epidermal cells) produce the protein keratin. When acne occurs, the dead cells that are located in your hair follicles are shed more frequently and in an abnormal fashion. Isotretinoin helps you to more normally shed away dead skin cells, so that they are less likely to clog your pores. This process prevents comedones (whiteheads and blackheads) from forming. I explain the formation of comedones and keratinization in Chapter 3.

Doctors usually prescribe isotretinoin after other acne treatments have failed to produce satisfactory results. Isotretinoin should never be the therapy of first choice. It must be demonstrated that you've been unresponsive to other standard therapies — the course of which usually begins with topicals (see Chapters 7 and 9), and moves onto oral antibiotics (or a combination of oral antibiotics and topicals, as I discuss in Chapter 10), or antiandrogens in women (see Chapter 11), all of which produce far fewer side effects than does isotretinoin.

Because of its serious side effects (see "Knowing What to Expect When You Take Isotretinoin" for more information), isotretinoin should be used only for severe, resistant acne. The drug isn't for everyone. However, when any of the following types of acne exist, isotretinoin may be considered (as the final therapeutic option):

- ✔ Severe nodular acne that can't be cleared up by any other acne treatments including oral antibiotics

- ✔ Inflammatory acne with scarring that has failed conventional treatment

- ✔ Moderate-to-severe acne with frequent relapsing

- ✔ Acne with severe psychological distress

I need to emphasize that those last three reasons to use isotretinoin are considered to be "off-label," meaning that the U.S. Food and Drug Administration (FDA) hasn't approved isotretinoin for these conditions. *Off-label use* doesn't imply that the drug is being used improperly or illegally. The decision to prescribe isotretinoin for the final three reasons has been based on many years of clinical experience and a careful consideration of the potential risks and benefits in the use of the drug.

 Isotretinoin can cause severe birth defects if taken by a pregnant female or a woman who becomes pregnant while taking the drug — even for a short time. Because the drug stays in the body's system for a long time, it can cause birth defects for one month *after* a woman has stopped taking it. Isotretinoin also carries an increased risk of miscarriage when used during pregnancy or up to one month prior to pregnancy. Studies done in males taking isotretinoin showed no significant effects on their sperm and no long-term damage to a male's ability to have healthy children.

Some of the birth defects include:

- ✔ Skull abnormalities
- ✔ Heart defects
- ✔ Deafness
- ✔ Cleft palate
- ✔ Central nervous system defects

In the treatment of females of childbearing potential, isotretinoin should be used only for patients with severe, disfiguring, cystic acne.

 If you have unprotected sex without birth control, miss your period, or become pregnant while you're taking isotretinoin, call your dermatologist immediately!

Preparing for Treatment

Isotretinoin's toxicity during pregnancy has long been known, but past efforts to reduce birth defects, including stricter product labeling and a limited pregnancy testing system, failed to resolve the problem. Therefore, in 2005, the FDA established an isotretinoin federal registry program called iPLEDGE. The program is geared toward reducing the number of birth defects, miscarriages, and abortions associated with the drug. The iPLEDGE program only applies to prescriptions for isotretinoin that are written in the

United States. But the precautionary information is valid no matter where you live, and many of the same procedures are followed throughout the world.

The registry keeps tabs on all isotretinoin prescriptions in the United States. Manufacturers, wholesalers, pharmacists, prescribers, and patients are linked through a centralized computer registry. The registry also connects to the laboratories that perform the required pregnancy testing in this system (see the next section, "Procedures all patients must follow," for details). Physician and patient identification codes are intended to protect the privacy of patients.

Unfortunately, some dermatologists and other healthcare providers, maybe yours, will stop prescribing isotretinoin rather than take on the time-consuming workload inherent in the iPLEDGE registry.

Note: In this section, I use the term *prescriber* to refer to the person who writes the isotretinoin prescription, whether it's your dermatologist or primary care provider.

Procedures all patients must follow

Everybody in the United States who is prescribed the drug, including females who can't get pregnant and males, must register with iPLEDGE.

The registration procedure requires your prescriber — or a designated person in your prescriber's office — to connect with the iPLEDGE Web site or phone system to enroll you into the system before being permitted to prescribe isotretinoin. Reactivation must be done on an annual basis. After you're registered and been prescribed isotretinoin, your prescriber must confirm to the registry that you are receiving ongoing counseling each month while taking the drug. A monthly review about birth-control requirements is especially crucial for female patients of childbearing potential (see the following section).

In addition to keeping tabs on all the prescriptions, registering everyone is meant to discourage men from sharing their isotretinoin with a girlfriend, sister, wife, and so on and to discourage women from asking men they know to get isotretinoin for them.

 Before starting treatment, your isotretinoin prescriber will order a lot of blood tests. A complete blood count, liver function studies, and triglyceride and cholesterol levels should be determined before treatment begins. That's because isotretinoin can cause changes in the blood and the liver. Your prescriber will likely continue to order more tests as treatment continues.

Your prescriber will also explain the risks and requirements for safely using the drug, and have you or your parent or guardian sign a consent form that says you understand the risks associated with isotretinoin, including possible birth defects as well as the possibility of depression and suicide. (Pharmacists must also hand out a detailed warning brochure.)

All patients, male or female, are only allowed a 30-day supply of isotretinoin at each office visit. These prescriptions are only valid for seven days after they're prescribed.

You must be reliable and capable of understanding the prescriber's instructions on the use of isotretinoin and the risks involved, and be willing to comply with these instructions.

Be sure to talk to your doctor about any of the following conditions that you or a family member may have:

- ✔ Allergies to foods or medicines
- ✔ Anorexia nervosa
- ✔ Asthma
- ✔ Diabetes
- ✔ Heart disease
- ✔ Liver disease
- ✔ Mental problems
- ✔ Osteoporosis

Additionally, tell your doctor if you're taking phenytoin (Dilantin), because using it in combination with isotretinoin may weaken your bones.

Additional steps females must take

Because isotretinoin is harmful to the fetus and therefore shouldn't be used during pregnancy, women of childbearing age must commit to additional testing and compliance in order to receive isotretinoin.

Table 13-1 contains a breakdown of the monthly responsibilities that you, your prescriber, and your pharmacist share within the iPLEDGE program if you're a woman capable of having children.

The discuss these requirements in the following sections (for more information you can check out www.ipledgeprogram.com and talk to your prescriber).

Table 13-1	Monthly iPLEDGE Requirements for Females Capable of Having Children	
Individual	_Interaction_
Your doctor	Confirms that you've received contraceptive counseling
	Enters the two types of contraceptives that you've chosen to use
	Enters your pregnancy test results
You	Answer educational questions before each prescription
	Enter the two types of contraceptives that you've chosen to use
Your pharmacist	Checks with iPLEDGE to get authorization to fill the prescription.

In addition to these steps, you also need to avoid becoming pregnant for at least one month after stopping isotretinoin treatment. And because of isotretinoin's potentially serious side effects, nursing mothers should unquestionably not use it.

Male patients who are taking isotretinoin should be informed about the risk associated with use during pregnancy, emphasizing that they shouldn't share the drug with females.

Birth control discussion

You must discuss birth control methods with your prescriber or a healthcare professional with expertise in contraception, such as a gynecologist. Such counseling and patient education are prerequisites to obtaining isotretinoin prescriptions.

Two negative pregnancy tests

Two negative pregnancy tests before you start isotretinoin are necessary. The first test (a screening test) is done when the decision is made to start isotretinoin. The second test (a confirmation test) must be done during the first five days of your menstrual period right before starting isotretinoin. You won't get your first prescription for isotretinoin until there is proof that you have had two negative pregnancy tests.

The pregnancy tests are performed only at certified laboratories that are CLIA approved. CLIA stands for Clinical Laboratory Improvement Amendments and was enacted by the United States Congress to ensure the accuracy, reliability, and timeliness of patient test results regardless of where the test was performed.

Ongoing pregnancy tests during treatment

You continue to have a pregnancy test every month during isotretinoin therapy. Along with confirming that appropriately timed initial pregnancy tests performed at a CLIA-approved laboratory are negative prior to authorizing the dispensing of an isotretinoin prescription for a female patient who is capable of becoming pregnant, the iPLEDGE registry requires a new pregnancy test before each refill is authorized.

Use of two separate forms of effective birth control at the same time

You must be using two of these birth controls at least one month before beginning therapy, during therapy, and for one month after isotretinoin treatment has stopped. Effective forms of birth control include:

- ✔ Hormonal birth control — including birth control pills, patches, long-term injections (like Depo-Provera), and implants (like Norplant)

- ✔ Condoms

- ✔ IUDs (or Intra Uterine Devices)

- ✔ Diaphragms

- ✔ Tubal ligation (having your tubes tied)

- ✔ A partner who's had a vasectomy

The following are unacceptable forms of contraception:

- ✔ Progesterone-only minipills that don't contain estrogen (In fact, if you're taking this form of birth control, talk to your doctor, as it may not work while you're taking isotretinoin.)

- ✔ IUD Progesterone T

- ✔ Female condoms

- ✔ Natural family planning (rhythm method) or breastfeeding

- ✔ Fertility awareness

- ✔ Withdrawal

- ✔ Cervical shield

Overcoming embarrassment

When she was a 17-year-old girl, Liza was prescribed isotretinoin, which she took for five months. Before starting the isotretinoin, she was asked by her dermatologist if she was sexually active or if there was any chance that she might be pregnant. She was also questioned about her knowledge about birth control methods. She was mortified because she was asked these questions right in front of her father!

After she began taking isotretinoin, she was embarrassed about having to go for the pregnancy test every month. I explained to her that it would have been irresponsible had the doctor not brought up the issue of pregnancy or if the doctor did not discuss birth control methods as well. Regrettably, these are embarrassing, but very necessary topics we must discuss because of the potential serious consequences that can occur if these issues aren't addressed and understood completely. Maybe her dermatologist could have been more tactful and spoke to her privately or asked her to bring her mother on follow-up visits.

As things turned out, Liza was very happy with the results of treatment and her worst side effect was really, really dry lips. "I went through four or five tubes of Chapstick," she said.

All birth control methods (besides *total* abstinence) can fail. Discuss the various options with your prescriber or your contraception advisor.

In two specific situations, you don't need to use these birth control methods:

✔ You commit to being absolutely and consistently *abstinent* (no sexual intercourse) during and for one month before and one month after your isotretinoin treatment.

✔ You have had a *hysterectomy* (your uterus was surgically removed).

If you are capable of becoming pregnant — even if you commit to abstinence — your prescriber may insist that oral contraceptives are one of the two methods used before starting, during, and for one month after isotretinoin treatment is completed.

Knowing What to Expect when You Take Isotretinoin

If I haven't scared you off yet with all the warnings earlier in this chapter, here's the section that tells you how to take isotretinoin, what to look out for, and how to deal with some of its inevitable side effects.

Taking your pills and observing results

Isotretinoin is available as capsules in the following strengths: 10, 20, 30, and 40 milligrams. The recommended dose depends on your body weight. Usually you take a pill with food twice a day for a total of 15 to 20 weeks. (In Europe, patients are often given lower dosages for longer periods of time.) Initially, your doctor may decide to start you off on a low dose so that you can get used to any side effects and then the dosage can be increased.

Often there is an observable improvement over the first month that continues over the course of treatment. In the vast majority of isotretinoin users, complexions smooth out, marks fade, and acne improves dramatically. Some lesions may still remain after you have stopped treatment, but many individuals notice that their acne continues to improve even in the weeks after treatment has stopped.

Shortly after starting isotretinoin therapy, some people may initially get worse before they get better. Often that's because they stopped all of the other acne medications that they were using up until then. A minority of isotretinoin users have a more serious flare at the beginning of treatment. Your dermatologist can manage this by adjusting the dosage or by adding other medications to calm things down.

Most people don't require a second course of treatment; when needed, it should be resumed only after the drug has been stopped for four months.

What not to do when you're taking isotretinoin

You must avoid certain things while taking isotretinoin, including the following:

- ✔ If you're a woman, don't even consider having unprotected sex while you're taking isotretinoin.

- ✔ Don't breastfeed while taking isotretinoin and for one month after stopping.

- ✔ Don't donate blood during treatment or for one month after stopping treatment. If someone who is pregnant gets your donated blood, her baby may develop severe birth defects.

- ✔ Treatment with tetracycline and isotretinoin shouldn't be given at the same time because the combination has been associated with brain swelling *(pseudotumor cerebri)*.

- ✔ Vitamin A should be strictly avoided while undertaking therapy with isotretinoin because they're closely related to one another. The use of both vitamin A and isotretinoin at the same time may lead to added side effects.

- ✔ If you're taking birth control pills, the herbal supplement St. John's Wort may make the birth control pills work less effectively.

Sizing up side effects

Although they're common, side effects with isotretinoin are usually tolerable. In general, most folks work through many of the reactions because the drug is so effective that people with severe acne want to continue taking it despite some of the bothersome side effects.

Side effects of isotretinoin are *dose-related*. That means that the higher the dosage, the greater chance of having side effects. One way around this problem is for your dermatologist to put you on a low dosage for a longer period of time. However, females will then have to continue monitoring pregnancy tests and continue birth control for a longer period of time.

Mild side effects

Isotretinoin is effective, in part, because it can shut down the oil production in the body, but this action accounts for some of its side effects. Because of the great decrease in oil production, even your mucous membranes, such as the inside of your nose, eyelids, and mouth, lose oil and become very dry. In fact, dryness is the most common side effect of isotretinoin. This reduction of oil can result in some of the less serious side effects, such as:

- **Dry lips:** Dry, chapped, and sometimes cracked lips are the most common and persistent annoyances from isotretinoin. These irritating problems occur in just about everybody who takes the drug. You can deal with them by gobbing on lip balm. I recommend Vaseline Petroleum Jelly, Chapstick, or Bag Balm.

- **Dry eyes:** You may find dry eyes to be a problem, particularly if you wear contact lenses. You may need to stop wearing them temporarily, but the frequent use of artificial tears such as Tears Naturale or Visine True Tears may allow you to continue using contacts. Artificial tears are used as one or two drops placed in the affected eye(s), as needed.

- **Mild nosebleeds:** Nosebleeds occur when the nasal lining dries out. They're usually short-lived and can be stopped with direct pressure. Nosebleeds can be prevented by coating nasal surfaces with lubricants, such as Vaseline Petroleum Jelly or Aquaphor ointment.

- **Dry skin:** You may notice peeling of your palms and soles, or scaly skin on the backs of your hands and forearms. Helpful moisturizers such as Eucerin cream, Moisturel, Cutemol, and Am-Lactin, are all available over the counter.

However, reduction in oil isn't the only annoying problem you face. You may also experience:

- **Aches and pains:** Musculoskeletal symptoms such as pain or stiffness of large joints or of the lower back occur and are usually very mild and disappear after a month or so. Try Tylenol (acetaminophen) if you experience ongoing pain.

- **Increased sensitivity to the sun:** I know you're all wearing sunscreen daily anyway (hint, hint), so apply it more often and use a higher SPF than you might normally.

- **Thinning hair:** Less common, but still annoying; some people have reported thinning hair during treatment. Rarely has this been a persistent or a permanent problem — the hair generally grows back when the treatment regimen is over.

A no-brainer

Roger was a 15-year-old when he first walked into my office with his parents. Before Roger came to my office, his family doctor called and told me that he had prescribed oral antibiotics and many creams and gels for Roger to try, but they did very little to improve his complexion. Roger's head hung low and he avoided eye contact with me. His face was studded with red papules, pustules, and acne nodules. He very reluctantly removed his shirt after I asked him to do so.

When I saw his chest and back, I then understood why he was hesitant to take his shirt off — his back and chest were covered with large acne cysts (nodules). Roger wasn't communicating much with me, but his parents told me that he refused to try out for his school swimming team even though he was terrific in the butterfly and backstroke. I guessed that he was ashamed to get undressed in the locker room because of the appearance of his skin. On top of all this, his parents said that his grades were falling off in school, he was sleeping later than usual, and that he stayed in his bedroom most of the time when he was home. All of these behaviors can be a consequence of his embarrassment about his appearance; however, they can also be indicators of depression, so Roger's parents were right to be worried about him. In Chapter 17, I point out the signs and symptoms of depression.

I also noticed that his dad had obvious acne scars on his face and he told me that he had pretty bad acne when he was a teen. He lifted his shirt and showed me that he was quite scarred on his chest and back. It was a no-brainer; Roger had severe nodular acne which, no doubt, would eventually heal and form scars just like his dad. After lengthy discussions with Roger and his parents, I ordered certain blood tests that proved to be normal and I prescribed a five-month course of isotretinoin for him.

To make a long story short, Roger's acne cleared up beautifully. One year after he finished taking the isotretinoin, he popped into my office with his girlfriend. He said that he just wanted to say "hi" and show me how great his skin looked. There were no scars! He did say that he would get a few pimples now and then, but he was able to control them with an over-the-counter medication. I asked him about the swimming team. Sorry to say, he tried out, but didn't make it. Well, maybe next year.

More serious problems

More serious unwanted events have also been reported and you should stop taking isotretinoin and call your dermatologist if you experience any of the following side effects. Most, if not all, of these side effects disappear after treatment is stopped, however, some have persisted after therapy:

> ✔ **Changes in mood, depression, or suicidal thoughts or attempts:** For more on this topic, see the section "The risk of depression and suicide."

✔ **Allergic reactions such as an itchy red rash or difficulty breathing:** In some people, isotretinoin can cause serious allergic reactions. Stop taking it and get emergency care right away if you develop hives, a swollen face or mouth, or have trouble breathing. Also stop taking isotretinoin and call your prescriber if you develop a fever, rash, or red patches.

✔ **Changes in vision:** You may experience decreased night vision. You should be particularly careful when driving at night. Rarely has this persisted following treatment.

✔ **Persistent headaches:** A rare side effect of this drug is benign intracranial hypertension, which is an increase in pressure of the fluid surrounding your brain. If you have continual headaches that are present in the morning on waking and wear off through the day, you should be evaluated by your doctor.

✔ **Hearing impairment:** This problem has rarely persisted following treatment.

✔ **Skeletal hyperostosis:** This condition is typified by excessive bone growth along the sides of the vertebrae of the spine. It is diagnosed by X-ray studies. This problem is limited to those who take a high dosage and long-term therapy with isotretinoin, a dosage much higher than is used to treat acne.

The risk of depression and suicide

Depression is unfortunately a common problem in the age group that needs isotretinoin most frequently — the adolescent group. Acne appears most often between the ages of 12 to 24. The onset of depression also commonly occurs at about the same time. In the United States, the FDA has been receiving reports of depression and suicide in patients taking isotretinoin and there is concern about a possible link between the drug, psychiatric disorders, and suicide.

Emotional problems in the adolescent population coupled with the stress of having severe acne, makes it difficult to determine whether isotretinoin can trigger depression and suicide or whether successful treatment may thwart such problems. This controversy has made its current use an issue of concern for many dermatologists and patients alike.

The package insert provided with isotretinoin prescriptions includes warnings about mental problems and suicide. Depression, other serious mental problems, suicidal thoughts, suicide attempts, and aggressive, violent behaviors have been reported while patients took the drug or soon after stopping it. No one knows if isotretinoin

Keeping yourself informed

If you're deciding whether or not to take isotretinoin, give it a lot of thought and do a lot of research. Check out the Internet, talk to your doctor, and read the information pamphlet that you were given by your dermatologist. The following are some Internet resources that you may find helpful:

✔ **FDA's Isotretinoin Information Page** (www.fda.gov/cder/drug/infopage/accutane/default.htm): The latest information from the FDA about isotretinoin.

✔ **Acne.org** (www.acne.org): A forum on which many people keep diaries on isotretinoin use.

✔ **Drugs.com** (www.drugs.com/MTM/isotretinoin.html): A good site for isotretinoin information.

✔ **Accutane/Roaccutane Action Group** (www.accutaneaction.com): People who suffered continuing side effects from Accutane and Roaccutane.

✔ **Chat group** (www.hayllar.com/accutane/archives/001736.html): Sarah's Accutane Journal.

caused these behaviors or if they would've happened even if the person didn't take the drug.

According to a recent study, isotretinoin doesn't cause depression. In fact, many patients in this study described themselves as being emotionally better off after being on the medication. Many dermatologists believe the research supports what they have seen in their patients all along. (If you're into medicalese, you can find the study by Christina Chia and her fellow researchers in the May 2005 issue of the journal *Archives of Dermatology;* http://archderm.ama-assn.org.)

One Canadian study found that 4 percent of patients taking isotretinoin became depressed and remained depressed during treatment with isotretinoin; however, there were no control subjects for comparisons. Studies of this sort, without controls (persons not taking isotretinoin), can't provide convincing scientific data about whether a common disorder — depression — is caused by a drug. The FDA currently regards these associations as unproven, but needing further study.

The bottom line, as of 2005, is that it is still unclear whether isotretinoin causes increased risk for depression and possible suicide. Because suicide is a major cause of death in teenagers, particularly in males, it has been difficult to determine a causal relationship between isotretinoin and these events and there is a great need for further study.

If you or your child is taking isotretinoin and is showing signs of moodiness, depression, or psychosis, the drug should be stopped and you should notify your dermatologist immediately so that the situation can be evaluated. In Chapter 17, I provide a list of depression warning signs, but also stop taking the drug and contact your doctor should you see signs of acting on dangerous impulses or seeing or hearing things that are not real.

Chapter 14

Searching for Weapons of Zit Destruction

*B*ecause of the concerns and debates over the safety of Accutane and long-term antibiotic use in the treatment of acne, lasers and other newer technologies that work on the surface of the skin will probably play an ever-larger role as future therapies for acne. In this chapter, I describe the use of lasers and other light sources in the treatment of acne and go on to tell you about what is known about treating acne with chemical peels.

You Light Up My Face: Zapping the Zits

Using lasers and light therapies offers a promising, noninvasive alternative to treat acne. Lasers and lights show evidence of improving not only inflammatory acne, but can also lead to improvement in acne scars. (See Chapter 16 for more information about scarring.) The long-term benefits of lasers and other light sources as methods for prevention and treatment of acne itself, is presently an open question, but the future appears bright. Until more is known, laser and light therapies may offer an alternative for people whose acne hasn't responded to traditional acne therapies.

Lasers can be tuned to target specific structures. When used to treat acne, the beams are adjusted to penetrate below the epidermis without causing any injury to it. They travel into the dermis where they can zero in on hair follicles, sebaceous glands, and the *P. acnes* bacteria (see Chapter 3 for more on the formation of acne). Certain lasers can also be used to destroy "broken" blood vessels (telangiectasias) in the dermis (see Chapter 18 for more on the telangiectasias); some lasers, by heating dermal collagen, can help to "tighten" the dermis and result in less visible scarring. Lasers that are used in acne scar treatment are the resurfacing (ablative) lasers and the non-ablative lasers, which are described in Chapter 16.

Researchers are hopeful that such treatments will lead to a reduction in the amount of drugs required to treat acne. At this stage of the game, laser and light therapy seem to be most helpful when used in combination with traditional acne medication treatments. Most acne patients using these technologies generally must continue to use topical and oral medications; however, several investigators report that some patients tend to require less oral and topical antibiotic treatments when lasers or lights are effective.

There are two basic groups of acne-treating lights. One group of technologies inhibits the growth of the bacteria *P. acnes* and the other group of light sources aims to shrink the sebaceous oil glands that also play a pivotal role in causing acne.

 Most insurance plans classify the light and laser treatments used to treat acne as "emerging technologies" and will probably not pay for your treatments. Many are still in the investigational stage and may not be the first choice for treating *your* acne. All of these treatments are expensive, time-consuming, and some are still in the experimental stage.

 Many people who have dark skin have been told that laser treatment is not safe for them. However, in expert hands, very specific wavelengths of lasers can minimize complications such as PIP (see Chapter 12 for more information) and scars.

Radio waves: Beam my acne away

Studies on radiofrequency emissions to heat up the sebaceous gland, tighten collagen, and shrink scars with pulses of electromagnetic energy are showing some promise. Currently, this technology is being used to tighten the skin as a noninvasive facelift. The radio waves heat the dermis without burning the surface. The surface is initially cooled with liquid nitrogen, after which a dosage of radio waves is applied. Definitely *stay tuned!*

Honing in on P. acnes with photodynamic therapy

Photodynamic therapy (PDT) involves applying a drug called a *photosensitizing agent,* which is then activated by exposure to a light source. Light sources used in PDT include visible (nonlaser) or laser light. This combined interaction of the solution and the light is what gives rise to the term "photodynamic therapy."

The U.S. Food and Drug Administration (FDA) has approved a non-laser, narrow-band, high-intensity visible blue-light therapy for treating inflammatory acne. It works by killing the acne-causing bacteria, *P. acnes.*

The *P. acnes* that reside in your sebaceous glands produce chemicals known as *porphyrins* as a by-product of their metabolism. Visible light — in this case blue light — seeks out the porphyrins that are in the bacteria. This high intensity light activates these porphyrins and thus kills the bacterial cells. Researchers hope that the sebaceous gland is "knocked out" or at least slows down as a result of this procedure (as a sort of "collateral damage"); however, we don't have hard evidence to actually document that this procedure succeeds in accomplishing it.

A doctor, nurse, or technician applies a clear, painless solution, aminolevulinic acid (ALA), to your skin. ALA is a potent, photosensitizing agent that increases sensitivity to light. It's left on your skin for 15 to 60 minutes and allowed to accumulate in target cells — the sebaceous glands. An intense, visible light source (usually a blue light) activates the ALA. This takes about eight to ten minutes. The chemical reaction that occurs produces heat and the bacteria are destroyed.

Immediately after this treatment, if you go out in the sun — even for a few minutes — you can develop a significant sunburn and peeling. For about two days after the photosensitizing agent is used, keep your face from being exposed to strong, direct light. Be sure to use sun protection.

Other side effects tend to be mild and include temporary pigment changes, swelling of the treated areas, and dryness.

Many treatments may be necessary to achieve satisfactory results. Because this type of therapy appears to target only one cause, *P. acnes,* the acne may not respond in the long run. That's because the destruction of these bacteria is only temporary; they revitalize rapidly, so ongoing treatments are necessary.

Banishing blemishes with warmth?

The latest on the zit parade to treat your acne is the heat-based, at-home acne treatment device known as Zeno. This pricey device sells for over $200 and has a costly tip that needs replacing after 90 treatments. It supposedly works by delivering heat to individual zits and killing the *P. acnes* bacteria that are involved in causing acne.

The gadget looks like a silver cellphone and is sold online from the company as well as by dermatologists, cosmetic surgeons, and other doctors without a prescription. Zeno uses controlled, low-level doses of heat that's delivered to individual pimples. The makers of Zeno claim that the device can "clear up a pimple in just hours."

Until more is know about this device, and it proves to be effective, how about a trip to Tahiti, or maybe save your do-re-mi by heating a spoon with hot water and applying it to individual zits?

Microdermabrasion, a technique described in Chapter 16, is a gentle way to exfoliate the surface of the skin. Recently, some investigators have found that PDT can be performed on a "short contact" basis. Using PDT after a light microdermabrasion allows for better penetration of the ALA.

A new photosensitizing agent, known as *lemuteporfin,* that seems to better penetrate the sebaceous glands, is now being investigated as a potential acne photosensitizer.

Looking ahead: Stopping oil at the source and other promising paths

For longer term results, it appears to be necessary to destroy the sebaceous gland as well as the bacteria. Various light sources are being tried in order to more deeply penetrate into the sebaceous glands. Technologies currently under consideration as potential acne treatment include

✔ **Intense pulsed light (IPL):** These devices are similar to lasers, but they use a wider range of wavelengths as opposed to only a single beam of light. They employ a broad band of visible and near infrared wavelengths of light that block out other wavelengths. Pulsed light can deliver hundreds or thousands of colors of light at a time. Pulsed light machines use "cut off" filters to selectively deliver the desired wavelengths. These wavelengths can be customized to reach the specific targets such as blood vessels or other skin components that are being treated.

IPLs can penetrate various depths into the skin, and by using longer wavelengths, they may able to affect the sebaceous glands' growth and activity. Long-term studies are necessary to see how effective they will prove to be.

✔ **Pulsed dye laser (PDL):** Results for acne have so far been inconsistent. This laser is "tuned" to a specific wavelength of light. It produces a bright light that is absorbed by blood vessels. This laser is also being used to improve the appearance of acne scars and is effective in removing the enlarged blood vessels associated with rosacea. I talk about PDL and acne scars in Chapter 16 and PDL and rosacea in Chapter 18.

✔ **Pulsed light and heat energy (LHE) therapy:** This treatment combines pulses of light and heat, which researchers believe target both *P. acnes* and the sebaceous glands, two of the main causes of acne.

✔ **Diode laser:** This laser uses infrared frequencies that are longer, invisible wavelengths. It appears to be effective on not only acne, but on the acne scars as well.

Avoiding ultraviolet light

There was a time that acne was routinely treated with ultraviolet (UV) lights. Acne sufferers would visit the dermatologist for their weekly dosage of sunburns from sunlamps. The results? It looked like they'd spent a long day at the beach — they'd be red and peeling for days afterward. The treatment did make acne look better for a time and may have had some benefit as a peeling agent. It also helped to blend skin tones and hide the acne lesions. But as we now know, repeated exposure to high intensity UV rays should be avoided. Frequent exposure to ultraviolet light can promote

Looking back: X-rays

Many years ago, dermatologists treated severe acne with weekly doses of superficial X-rays. The treatment dramatically reduced sebum production and often produced excellent degrees of clearing of some of the most difficult cases.

However, long-term consequences of this treatment included the development of thyroid and parotid cancers in many of the treated people. Needless to say, this type of treatment is no longer used to treat acne.

Sunning in moderation

If you don't have a personal or family history of skin cancer or if you easily tan, maybe the sun can work for your benefit. As some of you people who have excessively inflammatory acne have discovered, you may see a dramatic improvement of your skin during the summer, particularly if you spend more time outdoors when the days are longer.

This improvement is due to the blending of skin tones that a tan affords. Sunlight also has a drying effect on the skin that may dampen or shrink the activity of your sebaceous glands. Another probable mechanism may be the sensitivity to light of the chemical *porphyrins* that are part of the acne-producing *P. acnes* bacteria's makeup.

You still should consider the risks versus the benefits of sun exposure and think of it just as you might think of a medication. If you decide it's worth the risk, use the sun wisely.

aging of the skin as well as certain skin cancers. The light sources used to treat acne today don't contain UV light. For more information on UV light, the sun, and your skin, see Chapter 22.

As for the proponents of tanning salons, they contend that:

- ✔ Exposure dries up acne and improves its appearance.

- ✔ Using artificial tanning equipment, like beds and lamps, as well as natural sunlight, can protect you against some forms of cancer by increasing your vitamin D levels.

Dermatologists (including myself) believe that artificial tanning equipment, such as beds and lamps, should be avoided particularly if you are at higher risk of sun damage.

Taking It from the Top

Chemical peels have become popular as anti-aging, facial rejuvenation procedures; however, they're sometimes used to treat acne as well. In this procedure, a chemical acid solution is applied to your skin, causing the skin to peel off so that new skin can regenerate. Some of the peels have fancy names, extravagant prices, and are associated with overstated expectations. In fact, many of them are just gimmicky variations on the basic peels I describe in this section.

The peels work on wrinkles by loosening the glue-like substances that hold the dead cells on the surface of your skin together, causing them to peel off (exfoliate). This allows the skin to renew itself and thus lessen the appearance of fine lines and wrinkles and balance out skin pigmentation.

Chemical peels also produce a similar exfoliating action in your hair follicles where the sticky dead cells congregate and block your pores, causing acne breakouts. (Check out Chapter 3 where I describe how the cells adhere to one another and cause acne.)

Chemical peels are probably not effective for the treatment of inflammatory lesions of acne. They seem to work best in the elimination of blackheads and whiteheads (comedonal acne).

Peels for acne are generally superficial and less apt to cause complications such as pigmentary changes to the skin. Deeper peels, with stronger concentrations of acids, are sometimes used to treat acne scars. (See Chapter 16 for more about the physical scars of acne.) Superficial peels don't penetrate below the upper layers of skin and can sometimes also help to even irregular skin tones by lightening the dark spots of acne (see Chapter 12). Finding the treatment that is right for you depends on your skin type, the activity of your acne, your degree of scarring, and of course — as with all cosmetic procedures — your ability to afford it, because most, if not all, health insurance plans don't pay for them.

With chemical peels, persistent redness, permanent color change, and scarring are possible, especially with the deeper, high-concentration peels. Reactivation of cold sores has also been seen. Most importantly, if you or anyone in your family has a history of keloids or other types of significant scarring tendencies, these procedures are probably not for you.

Not only can peels reactivate cold sores, they can cause them to spread over your entire face. If you have any evidence of active herpes blisters, don't have any sort of peel (or microdermabrasion, regular dermabrasion, or laser abrasion).

It's important to protect your skin from the sun after any chemical peel. Ask your doctor to recommend a sunblock with both UVA and UVB protection, and apply it daily for at least four weeks after the treatment.

Occasionally, a topical retinoid such as Retin-A is used to pre-treat the skin by thinning the skin's outer layer. This preparation allows for deeper penetration of the chemical solution. The pre-treatment period may take up to a month before the chemical peel is actually performed. I cover Retin-A and the other topical retinoids in Chapter 9.

Chemical peels can be administered by a doctor, a nurse, or an aesthetician. Most states limit aestheticians to lower concentrations of these acids. The lower concentration peels that are much less potent than those used in doctors offices have little, if any, effect on acne.

Experiencing an AHA or BHA peel

The two most commonly used chemicals for peels are the alpha hydroxy acids (AHAs) and the beta hydroxy acids (BHAs). Procedures using these chemicals are commonly referred to as "lunch hour" peels because they're the mildest of the chemical peels and show few after-effects; some folks get them on their lunch hours and are ready to go back to work right away. Both of these acids are also found in many over-the-counter cosmetic products, such as moisturizers and sunscreens, but when a medical professional performs the peels, concentrations are much higher.

Lactic acid, a trendy AHA found in many over-the-counter products and prescription moisturizers, is hardly ever used for in-office peels. Lactic acid is not a "fruit acid" like other AHAs, because it comes from milk. See the sidebar "Cleopatra took it off the top," later in this chapter, for an at-home lactic acid treatment story.

The two most commonly used acid peels are

- **Glycolic acid:** Glycolic acid, an AHA, peels off dead layers of the skin and, typically, requires no downtime. These peels are performed every two to four weeks in a series of four to eight sessions.

- **Salicylic acid:** Salicylic acid, a BHA, is oil soluble and can therefore penetrate oil-plugged pores. When used as in-office peels, these treatments can hasten the response of acne to treatment by reducing the amount of sebum being trapped in your hair follicles. It is repeated at two- to four-week intervals. Typically, you combine this treatment with oral or topical acne medications. The over-the-counter use of salicylic acid is described in Chapter 7.

The application of AHA and Beta peels are relatively fast and simple. No sedation or anesthesia is required, because you only experience a slight stinging when the solution is applied. The treatment usually takes about 10 to 15 minutes, but the concentration of the chemical solution or the length of time of the treatment may vary. After treatment, apply generous amounts of moisturizer.

Cleopatra took it off the top

Back in 20 B.C. (before Clearasil), Cleopatra, with the help of her handmaidens, exfoliated at home by having her face soaked in sour milk. There's lots of lactic acid in milk.

Instead of going to your doctor's office, a spa, or floating down the Nile to the nearest chemist, you can do it yourself at home with at-home peel kits. Companies such as Chanel, L'Oréal, and Lancome now offer glycolic acid peel kits that are supposed to diminish blemishes, wrinkles, and spots. How effective are they? Not very. But if Marc Antony were still around, I'd like to ask him what his opinion was.

The skin remains slightly pink for a few hours to a day, but you can use makeup to cover it up, if you like. Minimize (or completely avoid) sun exposure until the skin is completely healed.

Trying out a TCA peel

Trichloroacetic acid (TCA) peels are sometimes used for lightening areas of pigmentation. TCA penetrates more deeply than AHA and BHA and creates more active peeling, especially at higher concentrations. This method also carries a greater risk of scarring. As a result, lasers and light therapies have mostly replaced these deeper peels for the treatment of acne and scars.

TCA peels are medium-depth peels and should only be done in a doctor's office or in an outpatient surgery center, because they produce deeper penetration and destruction of the skin and must be used with great caution. TCA peels often don't require anesthesia (because the solution itself has a numbing effect on the skin).

When the TCA is applied, you may at first feel a warm or burning sensation, followed by stinging. Following the application, the skin develops a "frosted" appearance within a few seconds and the treatment is diluted with cool water.

Significant swelling may occur depending on the potency of the TCA that was used. Swelling should diminish after the first week and the skin will generally heal sufficiently to resume normal activities in approximately seven to ten days.

You shouldn't have such a medium-depth peel if you have dark skin. Furthermore, wait at least a year or more after being treated with isotretinoin (Accutane) before having such a peel.

Chapter 15

Seeking Alternative Treatments

*A*lternative and complementary healthcare measures are gaining popularity. *Alternative medicine* refers to medicine that's used in place of conventional medicine. *Complementary medicine* is a treatment that is used in addition to conventional medicine. In this chapter, I explore treatments that are alternatives to the conventional approaches that are described in the rest of this book. I look back to the past (B.C. — Before Clearasil) and I investigate the present from the ashrams of Asia to the beauty counters at Bloomingdale's.

Does Alternative Medicine Work?

Although more research is needed to investigate the effectiveness and safety of alternative and complementary methods, some people with acne have described an improvement in their skin after taking certain herbs, undergoing acupuncture, and exploring mind/body relaxation techniques such as meditation, biofeedback, and hypnosis.

Right from the get-go I must tell you that the treatments I describe in this chapter are not ones I subscribe to. I'm presenting them for the sake of being as inclusive as possible and to let you know that they're out there. My medical views and opinions come from the traditional Western medical perspective that's based upon the scientific method and what is known as *evidence-based medicine*. The evidence-based method focuses on using the best available scientific evidence as a basis for devising treatments.

The clearing of acne by spontaneous remission may play a role in the popularity of some of these natural treatments; in fact, they may simply work by the *placebo effect*. A placebo is a substance or procedure that contains no medication or obvious physical delivery of energy. Instead, placebos simply reinforce a patient's expectation to get well. So if patients think they will get better by taking them, they do.

Placebo effects can be powerful, of course, but the potential benefit of relieving symptoms with placebos should be weighed against the harm that can result from relying upon — and wasting your money on — ineffective products and procedures.

Having said that, keep an open mind and I'll try to keep mine open too.

Exploring Traditional Chinese Medicine

The term *Chinese medicine* refers to a number of practices, especially acupuncture and herbal formulas. Chinese medicine has been practiced for over 4,000 years. The long-established concept has been that any illness is a reflection of an imbalance or blockage of energy or *chi* (pronounced chee), in the body.

One of the major assumptions inherent in traditional Chinese medicine is that disease is a loss of balance between *Yin* and *Yang,* the opposite poles of energy. Yin and Yang are the dynamic force of the Tao, constantly interacting with one another. Thus, in Chinese medicine, the physician will treat the underlying imbalance, not the symptoms of the disease itself.

Trying Chinese herbs

For thousands of years, Chinese formulas (along with Indian, Tibetan, and Japanese approaches) have been used to treat acne. Herbal medicines are the prevalent tools used by Chinese physicians to reestablish the balance of Yin and Yang, returning the body to a healthy, balanced state *(homeostasis)*. Both herbs and acupuncture (described in the next section) are methods intended to restore homeostasis.

Chinese herbalists usually don't prescribe one single herb for their patients. Herbal preparations are usually made by blending a variety of different herbs. The individual ingredients are weighed, combined, and then cooked into a souplike mixture and drunk like a tea. The mixture can be very foul tasting.

The problem with herbal medications is that it's hard to know exactly what's in them because there is no regulation regarding their contents. Herbs can be just as potent as a medicine you get from your pharmacy. There have been reports of severe toxic reactions, so you should be very cautious before trying anything that is untested.

For those of you herbalists or do-it-yourselfers, I list just a few of the ingredients that are sometimes used to treat acne. The various herbs are combined based upon the type of acne that is present:

- ✔ Flowers of honeysuckle, dandelion, chrysanthemum
- ✔ Fruit of forsythia, Cape jasmine
- ✔ Roots of scutellaria, platycodon, licorice, red sage, Chinese angelica, scutellaria, scrophularia, coptis, red peony
- ✔ Leaves of loquat
- ✔ Bark of moutan and mulberry trees
- ✔ Seeds of tangerine
- ✔ Bulbs of Zhejiang fritillaria

Modern research techniques have been done on very few of these botanicals; however, feverfew, a member of the chrysanthemum family, has been shown to have anti-inflammatory properties in the treatment of mild acne when it's applied twice daily for six weeks.

Sometimes, if the smell or taste of the herbal medicine is unbearable, you can take capsule or tablet forms of herbal medicines instead.

This method is supposed to work very slowly. Some of those who are very committed to herbal medicine have reported that if they persevere, the herbs will work as a preventative as well as a treatment of their acne. But many Western doctors — myself included — believe that the acne would have cleared on its own and that any successes had more to do with belief in the treatment itself than in its efficacy.

Let your healthcare provider or dermatologist know about any herbal products you're taking or considering taking.

Trying acupuncture for acne

Acupuncture is a traditional Chinese treatment often used to relieve pain. But many people have seen therapeutic effects by using it to stop smoking, lose weight, and to improve acne. Your *chi,* or energy, travels through the body by way of invisible meridians. Acupuncture works by using tiny needles to stimulate these pathways at specific pressure points in order to restore the balance between Yin and Yang.

Tiny sterile needles are inserted into the skin at specific points on your body. The needle is left in place or stimulated either by twirling it, by using a heat preparation known as *moxa,* or by an electric current. An acupuncturist may also prescribe an herbal formula for a person to take in addition to the treatment.

Although there have been no well-designed studies evaluating the use of acupuncture for acne, there have been several reports that *auricular* (acupuncture applied to the ear) and *electroacupuncture* (acupuncture delivered by an electrical current) therapies may have lessened the inflammatory component of acne. But, on the whole, acupuncture is an unproven acne treatment.

Going Natural: Herbs and Supplements Are All around You

You can find herbs, herbal remedies, and products infused with herbs just about anywhere these days. Health food stores, drugstores, your local market, even the cosmetics counter at the department store all have products that contain herbs and botanicals. In this section, I help guide you down the road to figuring out what herbs *might* actually be helpful for your kind of acne.

If you're interested in finding out more information about herbs, refer to *Herbal Remedies For Dummies* by Christopher Hobbs (Wiley). And check out the National Center for Complementary and Alternative Medicine (www.nccam.nih.gov), part of the U.S. National Institutes of Health, to find out the latest on herbal treatments.

My advice is to not ingest any herb or supplement without first discussing the matter with a qualified healthcare practitioner. Just because something is touted as *natural* doesn't mean it's *safe.*

Actually, natural means, "occurring in nature." By the way, cyanide and arsenic are found in nature and so are hurricanes, earthquakes, and tornados. So, I'd say that the label *natural* is virtually meaningless.

Besides, many of the so-called "natural" products also contain many other "unnatural" chemicals including preservatives, dyes, stabilizers, and fragrances. In fact, if a product was truly natural, you probably wouldn't want to use it anyway. It might not stay fresh; it might smell really bad, and it might not penetrate your skin where it has to do its work.

Fighting bacteria with botanicals

There is a budding interest to study plants that contain antimicrobial substances that may help eliminate *P. acnes* (the bacterial strain associated with acne — see Chapter 3 for its story), thereby potentially reducing inflammation associated with acne. Here are a few of the more promising candidates:

- **Tea tree oil:** Tea tree oil (derived from the tea tree plant native to Australia) has long been regarded as a topical antiseptic in Australia. A laboratory study found that certain active components of tea tree oil effectively slow the growth of *P. acnes.* The oil's proponents claim that even severe cases of acne have been shown to benefit from it.

- **Green tea cream:** This herbal treatment is derived from the medicinal portion of the green tea leaf. Its advocates believe that the leaf is as effective as benzoyl peroxide in treating acne (see Chapter 7 where I talk about benzoyl peroxide).

- **Calendula:** Commonly known as pot marigold, you can buy this popular ornamental plant for your garden at most nurseries in the spring. Its orange flowers can be made into tinctures, lotions, and creams. Acne suffers are encouraged to wash their skin with tea made from the flowers. If marigolds don't clear your acne, try planting them in your backyard.

Reducing inflammation with herbs

The following herbs have been considered to have general anti-inflammatory properties and claims have been made that they may be helpful in the treatment of acne:

- German chamomile
- Witch hazel

✔ Licorice root

✔ Flaxseed and flaxseed oil

✔ Black currant seed oil

✔ Evening primrose oil

✔ Echinacea

✔ Goldenseal

Some herbalists contend that certain compounds can help specific types of inflammatory acne:

✔ **Belladonna:** For people who experience flushes of heat to the face or who have inflamed pustular acne that improves with cold applications

✔ **Hepar sulphur:** For painful, pus-filled acne

✔ **Kali bromatum:** For deep acne, especially on the forehead, in persons who are chilled and nervous

✔ **Silicea:** For pustules or pit-forming acne

Herbs can be as toxic and dangerous as prescription drugs!

Herbs at the cosmetic counter

Many cosmetic counters make statements about the botanical and natural ingredients that are found in their products. A variety of vitamins, minerals, and herbs can be quite appealing to those who seek a natural treatment for their acne. Green tea has become a popular ingredient in many cosmetic and health products: moisturizers, cleansers, bath products, shampoos, toothpastes, and perfumes.

Finding a professional herbalist

Before ordering a concoction of herbs from the Internet or just picking up a bottle of herbs off the shelf in a health food store, you should get advice from a qualified herbalist. As with all alternative treatments, you should always have a degree of skepticism. But if you're interested in finding out more about traditional herbs, you might ask the people who work in the health food store or check out some of the following Web sites:

✔ In the United States: www.americanherbalistsguild.com and www.naturalhealthholistic.com

✔ In the United Kingdom:
www.ex.ac.uk/phytonet/bhma.html

✔ In Australia: http://nhaa.org.au/

✔ In Canada: www.ccnm.edu/about.html

Going natural with minerals and vitamins

For those of you who wish to try natural products, the mineral zinc and the B vitamin nicotinamide both are believed to have anti-inflammatory effects on acne. Their true effectiveness remains to be proven. Here's some further info on these possibly helpful items:

✔ **Topical zinc** is found in certain topical erythromycin ointments. It is possible, but not entirely clear, that the zinc oxide contained in the ointment may contribute to the effectiveness of the product. One such prescription product is Theramycin Z. Check this out in Chapter 9.

✔ **Oral zinc** may be an effective treatment for inflammatory acne. It's available over the counter.

Zinc may cause an upset stomach and nausea and it may decrease the absorption of various antibiotics including the tetracyclines.

✔ **Topical vitamin B3** is found in Nicomide-T cream and gel. They're both available over the counter.

✔ **Oral nicomide,** which is available only by prescription, contains vitamin B3 as well as zinc oxide, cupric oxide, and folic acid.

Checking Out the Ancient Art of Ayurveda

Ayurveda is practiced in India and is gaining popularity in the West. According to Ayurveda, all diseases are caused by poor internal organ imbalances and an improper diet. Dietary measures using quality herbs are stressed to reduce the severity of acne and also to prevent breakouts.

Ayurveda depicts three biological humors or energies called *doshas.* The three doshas are called *vata, pitta,* and *kapha.* For good health and well-being to be maintained, the three doshas within you need to be in balance. This means that a person needs to maintain his original doshic makeup through life as much as possible to maintain good health. Factors such as the dietary choices you make and the lifestyle you lead can cause one or more of the doshas in your prakriti to increase or decrease from its original level and create an imbalance. If this imbalance isn't corrected, you eventually lose your good health. That's why restoring balance is the central theme of the ayurvedic approach to health.

According to Ayurveda, acne is caused by the aggravation of all the three doshas. The primary aggravated dosha, however, is pitta. Pitta dosha symbolizes heat or fire in the body. Bad food habits such as eating white flour and white sugar products, and greasy, fried, and spicy food, together with stress, tension, polluted environments, and excessive use of chemicals, also aggravate pitta dosha. This aggravated dosha erupts on the skin as acne and pimples. Dietary rules are available in detail at www.ayurvedwebline.com.

The following are some suggested Ayurvedic acne home remedies:

- ✔ Drinking a half a cup of aloe vera juice, twice daily.

- ✔ Applying a paste of nutmeg and a little water to acne lesions and affected areas.

- ✔ Using orange peel face packs. The orange peels are pounded into a paste with a little water and applied to the affected areas.

- ✔ Drinking the Sunder Vati herbal preparation that includes ginger, Holarrhena antidysenterica, Embelia ribes, and Kampo.

Some Ayurvedic herbal products often contain high levels of heavy metals, which are considered unsafe.

Ayurveda methods have not been scientifically tested, so the jury is out.

Taking a Deep Breath: Aromatherapy

Aromatherapy is a branch of herbal medicine. It uses aromatic essential oils such as jasmine, orange, and rose, which are extracted from plants. The oils are either inhaled or applied directly on the skin. They're supposed to modify the immune system as well as promoting calmness and a sense of well-being. Aromatherapy has been reported to be helpful in treating acne, rosacea, and wrinkles through an ability to harmonize moods and emotions.

Some of these plant-derived essences are incorporated into bath products or used for inhalation. For example, ylang-ylang oil, derived from a fragrant tropical flower, has been used for many years in the tropics to induce feelings of tranquility and relaxation.

You can expect aromatherapy will smell good and — not much else! But if stress seems to make your acne worse, I guess you may see some improvement if you find the smells relaxing.

Considering Homeopathy

The word "homeopathy" comes from the Greek words *homoios* (similar) and *pathos* (disease). The first homeopathic principle states that anything that is capable of producing symptoms of disease in a healthy person can cure those symptoms in a sick person. Homeopathy uses a system that treats a disease by the administration of minute, micro-dosages of a remedy that would in large amounts produce symptoms similar to those of the disease.

The following are just a few of the numerous homeopathic treatment suggestions for acne:

✔ **Antimonium tartaricum:** This remedy claims to be helpful for acne with large pustules that are tender to touch.

✔ **Calcarea carbonica:** This remedy is supposed to help improve the skin's resistance to infection, especially in individuals with frequent pimples and skin eruptions, who get chilly with clammy hands and feet, are easily tired by exertion, and are flabby or overweight.

✔ **Hepar sulphuris calcareum:** This remedy may be indicated when the skin is easily infected, slow to heal, and painful eruptions like boils appear. The pimples are very sensitive to touch and slow to come to a head; eventually, offensive-smelling pus may form.

✔ **Pulsatilla:** This remedy can be helpful if acne is worse from eating rich or fatty foods, and aggravated by warmth or heat. It is indicated especially around the time of puberty, or when acne breaks out near menstrual periods.

✔ **Silicea (also called Silica):** This is intended for a person with deep-seated acne. Infected spots are slow to come to a head, and also slow to resolve, so may result in scarring.

✔ **Sulphur:** This remedy is meant for itching, sore, inflamed eruptions with reddish or dirty-looking skin.

Homeopathy's background

This type of medicine was developed in the late 1700s by Samuel Hahnemann, a German physician. Hahnemann theorized that if large doses of something caused a healthy person to show symptoms of a disease, then taking mini doses would act sort of like a vaccine, a harmless "clone" of the illness that might help that person fight that same disease. He believed that these treatments were intended to "balance" the body's "humors" by opposite effects.

You can find these items at your local health food store; select the remedy that most closely matches your symptoms. Treatment is taken by mouth in the form of tiny tablets, powder, granules, or liquids.

 There have been few studies examining the effectiveness of specific homeopathic remedies for acne. Homeopathic remedies are usually harmless, and its supposed "cures" are probably due to the natural healing tendencies of our bodies. However, if serious acne or an illness strikes you, it's best to see a conventional physician rather than a homeopath.

Practicing Mind/Body Medicine

Many teens and adults believe that stress can trigger and worsen acne outbreaks. I talk about stress and its relationship to acne in Chapter 6. The hormone cortisol, which is released in the body during stressed or agitated states, has gained widespread attention as the so-called "stress hormone." Excesses of this hormone are believed to worsen acne. If this is so, stress reduction techniques and relaxation therapies that reduce a person's cortisol could prove to be powerful ways to treat acne.

Psychological therapies, meditation, relaxation therapy, hypnosis, biofeedback, and cognitive imagery have made claims to have some success in treating acne. Mind/body techniques help to alleviate feelings of anxiety and depression. The measures described in the next section rely on the concept of the interconnectedness of the mind and body. As to whether people experience significant improvement of skin conditions, such as acne, is debatable.

Practicing yoga

Yoga is well known for helping a person deal with stress as well as creating "balance" in the body. Yoga has been reported to offer physiological benefits such as normalizing endocrine function, increasing immunity, and decreasing anxiety.

If you're interested in yoga, you can look in your phone book under topics like "yoga, exercise, workout, fitness" and anything else that seems appropriate to find a yoga class in your area. You can also look for information at www.yogajournal.com. Or if you'd rather try it at home first, look for a book or video in your local library. And definitely check out *Yoga For Dummies,* by Georg Feuerstein and Larry Payne (published by Wiley) and the *For Dummies* yoga DVDs.

Healthy practice . . . yes. Helps to clear acne . . . dubious!

Meditation: Contemplating nothing

Meditation is a way of soothing the body and the mind in a comfortable, quiet place, allowing troubling thoughts to leave the consciousness. The key element of meditation is "focusing" on either something, or nothing. The object is to clear the mind of distracting thoughts. Millions all over the world use this technique in order to reduce their stress levels. It's hard to evaluate results; however, the price is right! You don't need to buy anything to try this out on your own.

Here are some basic instructions for meditating:

1. **Find a quiet place to sit comfortably.** Use a cushion if you'd like.

2. **Close your eyes.**

3. **Breathe naturally.** Don't try to breathe extra deeply, or exhale strongly. Just breathe normally.

4. **Gently bring your attention to your breath and begin to think about something or nothing.**

   Choose *one* thing to think about when you're starting. Alternately, clear your mind of anything except your own breathing.

5. **Don't try to control your thoughts.** Let them come and go as they will. But instead of acting on them, just notice them. Feel sort of detached about them.

6. **Continue meditating for 20 minutes or so.** You may need to work up to this goal.

7. **When you're done meditating, take about a minute to slowly return to normal awareness.** Open your eyes slowly and wait a few minutes before standing, just to let your body return to full awakening.

If you're interested in finding out more about meditation, look for *Meditation For Dummies* by Stephan Bodian (Wiley).

Relaxing . . . yes. Helps to clear your acne . . . doubtful!

Biofeedback and cognitive imagery

Biofeedback is a technique in which an individual is trained to control certain internal bodily processes that normally occur involuntarily, such as heart rate and muscle tension. During biofeedback training, a technician helps a person perform a relaxation technique, such as *guided imagery,* while she's hooked up to monitors that measure her heart rate and muscle tension. Guided imagery involves the formation of mental pictures to promote a variety of favorable physical and emotional effects. This combination of biofeedback and cognitive imagery allows an individual to visualize and understand the bodily changes that occur when she changes from being tense to being relaxed.

There is no reliable scientific evidence that these techniques have any real impact on acne.

Hypnosis

Hypnosis is sometimes touted as being effective in the treatment for a variety of skin conditions including acne. As with the other mind/body techniques described here, hypnosis may also help to alleviate feelings of anxiety and depression that some individuals experience with this skin condition. Some researchers speculate that it can help an individual become more relaxed and, as a result, may positively influence the activity of hormones and the immune system (which may contribute to reduced inflammation).

There is no scientific evidence that hypnosis does much for acne.

Part IV
Dealing with Scars and Associated Conditions

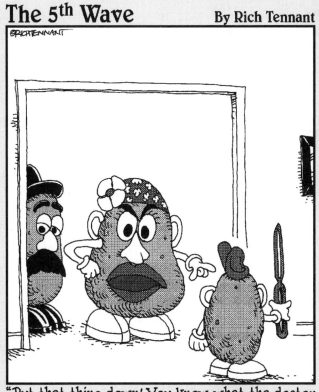

"Put that thing down! You know what the doctor said about picking at your skin!"

In this part . . .

I give you tips on how to treat acne scars based on the kinds of scars you have *and* the kind of skin you have. Because acne can be so emotionally devastating, I also delve into the emotional hurdles that you or your friends and family have to contend with and how to help avoid, manage, and prevent them. I then complete the picture with skin conditions that look like acne — the acne impersonators such as rosacea and razor bumps. I also tell you what symptoms may suggest an associated hormonal disorder.

Chapter 16

Focusing on the Physical Scars

. . . .

In This Chapter

▶ Figuring out what kind of scars you have

▶ Looking into whether you want to treat your scars

▶ Treating acne scars

. . . .

*T*he bad news is that acne can have lingering long-term effects — it can scar! The good news is that there are lots of ways to stop acne from scarring, and many of them are presented in this book. But if you *already* have scars, I have more good news — something can be done about them. In this chapter, I delve even more deeply into the dermatology tool chest in search of some heavy-duty and "light" tools that may help you with your acne scars.

The treatments described in this chapter are considered to be "surgical" in nature because they often involve cutting, abrading moving, building up, and destroying tissue (skin).

Examining Acne Scars

Acne scars are caused by the body's response — and sometimes, overresponse — to injury caused by inflammatory acne lesions. Most often, scarring results from severe nodular acne that occurs deep in the skin. But, scarring also may arise from more superficial inflamed lesions.

The term *scarring* technically refers to a process in which new collagen is laid down to heal an injury. *Collagen* is a protein that gives the skin its rigidity and strength and is produced by skin cells called *fibroblasts*. In Chapter 3, I talk about how scars are formed by collagen.

Scars can take on a number of different appearances: They may be flat; or sometimes, fibroblasts may work overtime and produce too much collagen that results in scars that bulge out like lumps. They can also form indentations (or pits) when there's a loss of skin that is replaced by collagen. Scars can be skin colored, whitish, purple, red, or even darker than a person's normal skin color.

There are times when "scars" aren't really scars. After an acne lesion has healed or even while healing, it can leave a pink, red, purple, or a darkly pigmented mark on your skin. These marks are actually *macules,* spots that indicate a *temporary* color change of the skin. These areas of remaining inflammation or post-inflammatory change aren't scars because no permanent change has occurred.

Sometimes, especially in darker-skinned people, the spots tend to be darker than the normal skin color and they tend to hang around longer. This is known as *postinflammatory hyperpigmentation* (PIP), an after-effect from a healing acne lesion itself. These lesions also tend to fade in time, unless the pigment winds up deep in the dermis *(dermal melanosis).* Dermal melanosis is a type of PIP that is much harder to treat and may never fade away completely. I cover PIP and options for stepping up the speed at which these lesions fade in Chapter 12.

Some people endure their acne scars all their lives with little change in them. Other people are luckier — their skin improves and the scars undergo some degree of improvement over time, and they sometimes transform *(remodel)* themselves and decrease in size. I guess time does heal some, if not all, wounds.

I characterize the different types of scars next. Keep in mind that some people have a combination of different types of scars so that one treatment may not work on them all.

Pulling in: Scars caused by loss of tissue

Some acne scars appear as holes, pits, or craters in the skin. Called *atrophic scars* or *crateriform scars,* these depressed, cavity-like, inward-directed scars are associated with a lack of tissue that occurs when the inflammation from healed acne causes destruction to the skin (similar to scars that often result from chickenpox). The scar tissue contracts and binds the skin down.

Terms and descriptions related to this type of scarring will be help-ful when talking with your dermatologist and reviewing treatment options, because some treatments work better than others for different scars. Here are some more descriptive names:

- ✔ **Ice-pick scars:** These scars are the most common acne scars that occur on the cheeks. They're most often small, with a somewhat jagged edge and steep sides — like wounds from an ice pick. They can be shallow or deep. Ice-pick scars may evolve into depressed fibrotic scars over time.

- ✔ **Depressed fibrotic scars:** These scars are usually quite large, with sharp edges and steep sides.

- ✔ **Boxcar scars:** These scars are angular and usually occur on the temple and cheeks, and can be either superficial or deep. They are similar to chickenpox scars.

- ✔ **Rolling "hill and valley" scars:** These scars give the skin a wavelike appearance. They have gently sloping rolled edges that merge with normal skin.

Growing out: Collagen running amok

Scars that bulge out and look like lumps are associated with an exaggerated formation of scar tissue due to excessive amounts of collagen production. These are the two most common of this type:

- ✔ **Hypertrophic scars:** These scars bulge outward like lumps.

- ✔ **Keloids:** A keloid is a scar whose size goes far beyond what would be expected from what seems to be a minor injury. It's kind of an "over-scarring."

You can see examples of both of these scars in the color section of this book. Both hypertrophic scars and keloids occur more commonly in dark-skinned individuals. They also tend to run in families — that is, growth of scar tissue is more likely to occur in people whose relatives have similar types of scars.

These scars persist for years, but may diminish in size over time. They're notoriously difficult to treat and impossible to completely eradicate. A single, optimal treatment technique for hypertrophic scars and keloids hasn't been developed, and the recurrence rate of these scars after treatment is high.

Surgical management is reserved for cases that are unresponsive to a conservative treatment, such as injecting cortisone into the scars themselves. The cortisone injections often help to shrink thickened, raised scar tissue. This procedure is similar to the procedure that is used to treat acne nodules that I explain in Chapter 10. Surgical treatment is a last resort because any person whose skin has a tendency to form these types of scars from acne damage may also form larger scars in response to any type of aggressive skin surgery. In some cases, the best treatment for keloids in a person who is highly likely to develop them is no treatment at all.

Certain lasers as well as *intense pulsed light* (IPL) devices that I describe in Chapter 14 may prove to be effective for these stubborn scars, but long-term studies are necessary to see how effective they will prove to be.

Taking Initial Treatment Steps

The oral and topical treatments used to treat acne don't do very much to improve the appearance of acne scars. However, dermatologists and plastic surgeons *do* offer a number of treatment options if you have scars. The type of treatment you decide upon should be the one that is best for you in terms of your type of skin, the cost of the treatment, and what you want it to accomplish.

Deciding whether you want to do anything about it

A decision to seek treatment for acne scars, and the specific treatments that you may choose, depend on a number of factors that you and your doctor can discuss and weigh:

- ✔ **How do you feel about your scars?** You may have scars and could care less about them or they may be psychologically distressing to you. Do the scars emotionally affect your life? Are you willing to live with your scars and wait for them to fade over time?

- ✔ **What's your age, overall health, and medical history?** If you're a teenager or healthy adult, you'd probably want to wait until your acne is no longer active. If you're an adult or senior who has medical problems and are taking several medications, consult with your primary care provider before embarking on any surgical procedure.

- ✔ **How bad are your scars?** Are they disfiguring? The severity of the scars can affect whether you're willing to go through treatment.

- ✔ **What kind of scars do you have?** Some scars respond more readily to treatment, and others, like keloids, indicate that treatment could actually cause more scarring.

✔ **What's your doctor's opinion?** An expert opinion as to whether scar treatment is justified in your particular case may help you decide upon the most effective treatment for you.

✔ **What do you want to accomplish?** Maybe you just want to diminish the appearance of deep scars or maybe you're trying out for a part in a feature film.

✔ **How will you pay for treatment?** Get a handle on your finances and insurance coverage before you make any decisions. You need to determine the costs that you'll have to pay out of pocket and whether you can afford to do so. A significant investment of time and money is often needed.

Most of these procedures aren't covered by health insurance plans because they're generally considered to be cosmetic in nature. It may go without saying, but I'll say it anyway: They're all pretty expensive. Just to give you an idea, a laser skin resurfacing can cost from $4,000 to $5,000 or more!

Also be aware that acne scars are particularly difficult to treat and they can't always be effectively corrected by one single treatment method. In fact, using more than one method may yield better results. Before committing to treatment of acne scars, you should have a discussion with your doctor.

Finding a physician

When you turn your attention to the treatment of acne scars, it's especially important that you find a doctor who is trained and experienced in the procedures that I describe in this chapter, for a number of reasons:

✔ Many of the treatments have sometimes been offered by inadequately trained practitioners, sometimes with devastating, disfiguring results.

✔ Some of the treatments may result in more scarring if you have a propensity to develop hypertrophic scars or keloids. You need a reputable, experienced physician to help you weigh the pros and cons with this type of scarring.

With the exception of microdermabrasion and most chemical peels, which can be performed by a physician, nurse, or licensed aesthetician, the procedures described in this chapter are performed by a dermatologist or plastic surgeon in her office.

If your doctor or dermatologist doesn't treat acne scars, check out Chapter 8 where I tell you how to find a dermatologist who does. You can also go to the Web sites of The American Academy of Dermatology (www.aad.org) and The American Society for Dermatologic Surgeons (www.asds-net.org). These sites can help you locate a dermatologist who has specialized training in cosmetic and other types of skin surgery.

To find a plastic surgeon who performs these procedures, visit the online referral service of the American Society of Plastic Surgeons (ASPS) at www.plasticsurgery.org. This is the largest plastic surgery organization in the world and the foremost authority on cosmetic and reconstructive plastic surgery. (Check out Chapter 21 for more online resources.)

Treating Your Scars

Don't start any treatment for scarring until your acne is *completely gone* and unlikely to come back. If you go to all the trouble and expense to undergo a procedure (or multiple procedures) and then get more acne, and thus more scarring, you have to go through it all again. Just imagine how expensive that would be!

Skin resurfacing techniques (like dermabrasion), surgical excision, and fillers have been used to diminish acne scarring for years with mixed results. Currently, laser therapy has assumed a more important role in the treatment of acne scars, and other newer surgical methods featuring light and radio waves are an option to treat your acne.

Most scar treatment focuses on facial scars. Generally, scars on the chest and back don't respond as well to the treatments mentioned hereafter. Because these scars are so hard to treat, the best approach is to try to prevent them in the first place. If the prevention route fails, the intralesional cortisone (steroid) injections that I describe in the "Growing out: Collagen running amok" section, earlier in the chapter, may help to shrink them.

One remnant of the recent past in treating acne scars is the chemical acid peel. Peels are sometimes used in the treatment of acne and dark spots (see Chapter 13), and you may still hear about them in conjunction with treating shallow acne scars. But, for the most part, the results of chemical peels in treating scars are disappointing, and the method has been replaced by others, notably lasers, that I discuss.

Laser skin resurfacing

There are many types of lasers and there are a number of new procedures now available that complement or even surpass previous scar revision techniques such as those that I describe later in the chapter. Treatment with some of these devices can be used to help improve and treat acne itself (see Chapter 14 where I discuss other types of lasers that treat acne in more detail), and as a simultaneous benefit, they can stimulate collagen remodeling and result in the improvement of the appearance of acne scars.

Laser resurfacing can result in uneven skin tones in people with darker skin.

Treatment with laser resurfacing takes place in an office setting. Typically three sessions are performed. For a "full-face" resurfacing, the cost can be $3,000 to $8,000 and up!

Sometimes, laser resurfacing and other surgical treatments (described in the "Considering other surgical treatment options" section) for acne scars are combined. The surgical treatment is usually completed 6 to 12 weeks before the laser is called into action. This waiting period gives your skin time to heal and remodel itself.

The two major categories of lasers that are used in acne scar therapy are the resurfacing (ablative) lasers and the non-ablative lasers.

Ablative lasers

The powerful ablative lasers literally remove the outer layers of the skin by using high-energy light to burn away scar tissue, and stimulate the dermal collagen to tighten, reducing the amount of scar visibility.

This procedure is used for deeper scars and carries the risk of further scarring. Because the skin is injured and unprotected tissue is exposed, great effort must be put into post-operative wound care and infection prevention. The skin may remain reddened for several months or a year afterwards.

Non-ablative lasers

At first, ablative lasers were used to recontour or vaporize the skin's surface. Now, techniques involving non-ablative lasers have taken over because of their ability to promote collagen growth beneath an acne scar without creating an external injury. The non-ablative lasers produce a controlled injury to certain target structures in the dermis, while completely sparing the epidermis from damage.

The laser beams can penetrate into the dermis without injuring the epidermis. By heating dermal collagen, they help to "tighten" the dermis and result in less visible scarring. The theory is that the thermal injury caused by the laser triggers a wound repair response, including fibroblast activation and new collagen formation.

Non-ablative laser resurfacing can be effective for treating shallow boxcar scars, as well as for smoothing and tightening scars that have been treated previously. It is not very effective for deep, depressed, craterlike scars.

A topical anesthetic is applied by a doctor or his medical assistant about an hour before performing these procedures to make the pain tolerable. The surface of the skin is cooled to prevent the laser from damaging the epidermis. A patient will feel both the cold spray as well as some amount of stinging and heat during the session.

Shooting scars

Non-ablative lasers include:

- ✔ **InfraRed Lasers** produce invisible light. They're most commonly used for thermally induced dermal remodeling and use water as their targets. They are minimally absorbed by *melanin,* the epidermal skin pigment, which makes them suitable for all skin types. These lasers use aggressive skin cooling to limit the heating effect, creating a controlled injury to the dermal collagen, with subsequent remodeling and tightening.

- ✔ **N-Lite Laser** is another non-ablative laser. It is now being used to trigger collagen formation.

- ✔ **Sprinkling laser beams:** A kinder, gentler laser is now available. This latest laser is called the Fraxel laser. Unlike older lasers, which shoot a single solid beam of light, the Fraxel laser shoots out tiny clusters of beams that burn the skin in patterns of dots. It burns away old skin cells and spurs the growth of new cells and stimulates the production of collagen that, in time, tends to "fill the dots" and smooth out the skin.

The theory behind this is that such "fractional" treatment allows the skin to heal much faster than if the entire area were treated at once, using the body's natural healing process to create new, healthy tissue to replace skin imperfections. There is less injury to the skin with this method and less downtime compared with the older lasers, and there's minimal discomfort as compared to the ablative lasers.

Considering other surgical treatment options

Atrophic scars, such as ice-pick scars, boxcar scars, and small depressed fibrotic scars, may be removed or improved by a *punch excision* of each individual scar.

Excising scars: When zits are literally the pits

In this procedure, each scar is cut down to the layer of subcutaneous fat; the resulting hole in the skin may be repaired with sutures or with a small skin graft. Alternatively, the punch may simply be elevated. There are three techniques:

- ✔ **Punch excision:** Your doctor removes the pitted scar with a cookie-cutter-like tool that punches out small portions of skin. The surrounding healthy skin is joined together by suturing.

- ✔ **Punch replacement:** As with the punch excision, the scar is removed and then replaced with a skin graft of unscarred skin, usually harvested from behind the ear. This method is usually the most successful for treating deep scars.

- ✔ **Punch elevation:** Here the scar is punched out, but not discarded. It is allowed to float up to the level of surrounding skin.

Your dermatologic or plastic surgeon may allow the scar from punch techniques to fade on its own. Or she may perform the procedure before a more generalized resurfacing technique such as laser resurfacing is performed. Less commonly, dermabrasion, microdermabrasion, and chemical peels are sometimes used in conjunction with punch techniques.

The prices of these procedures vary and depend upon the number of grafts or punches that are done. Punch grafting can run $50 to $150 per graft or $1,000 to $2,500 per session.

Subscising scars

Subcision helps to restructure and remodel scar tissue by breaking fibrous bands that are creating tension between the epidermis and deeper structures. It also helps induce new collagen formation. This method is useful for indented, rolling scars that result from scar tissue holding the skin down. This is a very specialized procedure that is performed by a qualified dermatologic or plastic surgeon.

To perform this technique, a sharp instrument such as a tiny scalpel or needle is used to undercut and lift the scar tissue away from unscarred skin, elevating the skin to make it even. The sub-scising procedure breaks down *adhesions* (old bands of scar tissue), which helps to reorganize the formation of new collagen and elastic tissue for a smoother skin surface. The overlying skin isn't cut, so sutures aren't needed.

This breaking down of scar tissue helps to level the playing field. After the wounds heal, an injection with a filler material under the scar can help to replace any remaining defects and bring them to surface level. The filler can be made of one's own fat or a collagen or other synthetic substance that I describe in the section "Contouring the defects: Fill 'er up!"

The procedure can cost between $200 and $1,000 depending on the number of lesions treated.

Contouring the defects: Fill 'er up!

Another option for improving the appearance of certain acne scars is known as *soft tissue augmentation*. These procedures have a very limited use, and at most, they can help with some of the shallow "hill and valley" soft scars with gentle sloping edges. They don't work well for ice-pick, deep boxcar, or depressed fibrotic scars.

Materials, including your own fat, can be injected into the depressed area of the scar to elevate it to the level of the normal surrounding skin. The material is injected under the skin to stretch and fill out superficial and deep "soft" scars. Many substances are available and many new ones continue to be introduced. Most doctors have a variety of fillers to choose from, including the following:

- **Collagen:** Collagen injections are intended to replenish your natural collagen and minimize surface unevenness by lifting and filling depressed lines and scars. The original bovine collagens Zyplast and Zyderm can't be used in people with autoimmune diseases. Skin testing to look for possible allergic reactions is necessary before they're injected.

  The newer human-derived collagen products such as Cosmoderm and Cosmoplast offer alternatives to those who are allergic to the bovine derived collagen. No skin testing is required with these agents.

  Collagen injections are temporary, and last about six months (give or take a few months), so ongoing touch-ups are necessary.

- **Fat:** To correct deeper defects caused by scarring from nodular acne, fat transplantation utilizes your own fat. The fat is taken from another site on your own body and injected beneath the surface of the skin to elevate depressed scars. Because the fat is reabsorbed into the skin over a period of 6 to 18 months, the procedure usually must be repeated.

✔ **Newer fillers:** There has been an increase in the number and quality of filler substances used to help plump up acne scars. Restylane and Hylaform are now available and there are many more to come. Longer-lasting results are expected from these materials.

Unless the borders of atrophic scars are soft, there is little place for fillers in the treatment of acne scars. They're probably best used as a complementary procedure with other surgical treatments described in this chapter. Depending on the type and amount of filler used, treatment can cost between $400 and $750 and $1,000 and $1,200.

Trying out dermabrasion

Before there were lasers, superficial acne scars were smoothed out with a procedure known as *dermabrasion*. Dermabrasion was used to minimize small acne scars. As the name implies, dermabrasion involves removing the top layers of skin.

Dermabrasion has been around for many decades. Initially, sandpaper was used to remove damaged skin and allow new skin to grow in its place — yes, I'm serious. But now, electrical machines are used to abrade the skin. These gadgets have quickly rotating wheels that have a rough wire brush *(fraise)*, or a burr containing diamond particles. The wheel is attached to a motorized handle.

Dermabrasion may make ice-pick scars and depressed fibrotic scars more noticeable if the scars are wider under the skin than at the surface. Dermabrasion is used mainly for the "softer" scars. It's rarely used for hypertrophic scars. Over the past decade, this procedure has fallen out of favor with the availability of newer, easier-to-use techniques such as lasers. I no longer recommend it.

A qualified dermatologic or plastic surgeon performs dermabrasion on a single visit as an office procedure. First she anesthetizes your skin with a numbing spray, such a Freon. You may also be given a sedative to make you drowsy before she sheers away your scar tissue. A full-face dermabrasion can be as costly as a laser resurfacing procedure. It can cost $2,500 to $4,500.

In darker-skinned people, dermabrasion may cause dramatic changes in pigmentation and worsen hypertrophic or keloidal scars.

Vacuuming your skin: Microdermabrasion

This technique is a surface form of dermabrasion. I call it "dermabrasion lite." Rather than a high-speed brush, microdermabrasion uses aluminum oxide crystals passing through a vacuum tube to remove surface skin. The crystals are literally blasted onto the skin and then vacuumed away accompanied by surface skin cells. Microdermabrasion can be performed by anybody — your Aunt Gertrude, a physician, a nurse, or an aesthetician.

At most, microdermabrasion is effective in reducing fine lines, "crow's feet," and age spots, but this treatment isn't effective for diminishing acne scars. That's because only the very surface cells of the skin are removed and a mild exfoliation takes place. Microdermabrasion runs from $150 to $300 per treatment.

Dermabrasion may result in pigmentary streaking in people with dark skin types. If you have dark skin, make sure your doctor has extensive experience (and success) at treating others with your skin type.

Considering emerging technologies

Many technologies that were initially developed as anti-aging wrinkle treatments are now becoming useful in treating the scars associated with acne, including radio waves. This novel treatment, referred to by the brand name Thermage, uses radiofrequency (RF) emissions to deliver controlled amounts of energy (heat) into the collagen layers of the skin. It has a cooled application tip to protect the epidermis from heating up. It's supposed to penetrate deeper in the skin than other methods and cause thermal injury to sebaceous glands. Currently, it's being used to tighten the skin as a non-invasive face-lift. More research is needed to see if it works on acne and acne scars. The procedure can cost between $2,000 and $5,000. See Chapter 14.

Chapter 17

Coping with the Psychological Scars

*T*he psychological impact of acne can lead you to feelings of diminished self-esteem and be a source of anxiety when it comes to dealing with the world. If you're a teen with acne, you may have been told, "It's no big deal, and anyway, you'll grow out of it. You're just experiencing a normal part of life." But to you, having acne *is* a big deal; you feel insecure and lack self confidence. Every day you have to deal with school and other kids who seem perfect (even if they're not). You don't feel like you have time to "grow out of it."

The truth is that many folks *don't* "just grow out of" acne and others wind up growing *into* it. And if you're an adult, you don't even get the benefit of having lots of other peers around in the same boat. You have a whole different set of stressors (job interviews, presentations, black tie events, and carpools) associated with your acne. And darn it, you thought you were past this stage anyway.

The main thing to remember, whatever age you are, is that acne is treatable. (Take a look at Chapters 7 through 15 to find just the right way to treat *your* acne.) In this chapter, I talk about ways to deal with the *invisible* scars that some people carry around with them — the ones that are carried on the inside. Although most other people see acne only on the surface, the burden goes much deeper.

Facing Acne Can Be Tough — But You Can Do It

Our society places a great emphasis on physical appearance. In a culture where looks are overly emphasized, feeling good about yourself is easier said than done. We're constantly bombarded with advertising that displays models and movie stars, all of whom are depicted as paragons of beauty and flawless perfection. They often serve as the spokespeople for health and beauty aids that imply that you can look like them if you "get with it" and do what they do or buy the products they're promoting.

When you see media portrayals of all those people with perfect skin, just remember that almost all of those photos are touched-up and airbrushed. Some of the models even have acne, just like you!

Even mild cases of acne can leave a person with a negative self-image — sometimes well beyond the degree of the actual physical appearance. These negative feelings are particularly prevalent when you have a concentration of lesions on your face, which is your greeting card and introduction to the world. Unlike many other skin conditions, acne lesions wind up on areas that often aren't concealed by clothing.

Acne is often a source of anxiety that can impact your self-image and confidence. Some of the things you might be experiencing are:

- ✔ Feeling uncomfortable in social settings
- ✔ Having less self-confidence
- ✔ Becoming more preoccupied with your appearance
- ✔ Feeling like you're trapped in a perpetual adolescence
- ✔ Being sad and sometimes getting depressed (see the following sections)

These negative effects and feelings can put pressures on your social, work, or school life.

Here are some suggestions that you can use to cope with some of these negative feelings:

- ✔ Wash your face no more than two to three times a day (unless you're a coal miner!). Check out Chapter 2 for my face washing tips.
- ✔ Get a new haircut or hairstyle (bangs are great!).

> ✔ Spruce up your wardrobe.
>
> ✔ Educate yourself. Read about acne in this or other sources.
>
> ✔ Find the right dermatologist or healthcare provider to treat your acne. (In Chapter 8, I tell you how to go about it.)

Here are some tips for if and when you start undergoing treatment:

> ✔ Stand at least two feet away from all mirrors for the next two months.
>
> ✔ Measure progress monthly instead of daily; be a patient patient!
>
> ✔ Take a picture of your acne when it's at its very worst. Put the picture in your bottom drawer and don't look at it for two months, because that's how long it may take to see significant improvement.
>
> ✔ Be sure you know the names of and exactly how to use your acne medications. (I spell out all of this information in Chapters 7 through 13).
>
> ✔ If you're still feeling emotionally overwhelmed and possibly depressed, see the next section.

Detecting Depression in Yourself and Your Family

It's very normal for people with severe acne to feel down and despondent; even mild acne can give you the blues. However, if you or someone in your family is feeling unhappy more often and doesn't seem to enjoy anything anymore, you need to consider the possibility that you or that person may be suffering from depression. Here are some of the signs of depression:

> ✔ Increased fatigue, low energy
>
> ✔ Feelings of pessimism
>
> ✔ Loss of enjoyment in things that previously gave pleasure
>
> ✔ Crying spells
>
> ✔ Sleep disturbances
>
> ✔ Hating to get out of bed
>
> ✔ Social isolation
>
> ✔ Loss of appetite or the opposite

✔ Lots of new physical complaints

✔ Decrease in sexual drive

✔ Irritability, anger, or aggressiveness

✔ Feelings of worthlessness and guilt

✔ Withdraw from family and friends

✔ Suicidal thoughts

If one or more of these descriptions rings a bell, talk to your doctor about it. If you or your loved one is having suicidal thoughts, seek immediate evaluation and treatment.

Helping Your Child Deal with Acne

Acne affects adolescents at a time when they're developing their personalities and evolving into adulthood. During this time, peer acceptance is very important to them and physical appearance and attractiveness is highly associated with peer status. Besides the physical scars that severe acne can produce, your teen may also be suffering emotionally.

Acne can be a real drag on a kid's daily life. Acne on the face can bring out cruel taunts, teasing, and name calling from other kids. Some kids become so preoccupied with how their skin looks, that they may not want to go to school, lose self-confidence, pull away from their friends, show a dramatic change in their thinking and behavior, become withdrawn, and even may begin to feel depressed.

The following list goes over some of the various teenage behaviors and coping mechanisms that they may develop to deal with acne:

✔ Grow their hair long to cover their face.

✔ Become so embarrassed that they avoid eye contact.

✔ "Cake on" heavy makeup to hide the pimples.

✔ Lose interest in sports such as swimming or basketball because of the need to undress in locker rooms and expose their back and chests.

✔ Become shy and even isolated and prefer to stay in their bedrooms.

✔ Start to develop any of the symptoms of depression from the list in the "Detecting depression in teens" section.

Offering your help

Here are a few seemingly simple, yet effective, ways to communicate your willingness to help:

- ✔ **Let your children know how much you care:** Give your child adequate time to bring up the subjects of their acne and allow them to address or respond to your questions about the behavioral changes you've noticed.

- ✔ **Listen patiently:** They may want to communicate their feelings but have difficulty doing so. Think back to your own teen years. You may not have always felt like it was easy to be open about your thoughts and feelings.

- ✔ **Don't be overly judgmental about your child's appearance:** Approach the subject of acne in a gentle, caring manner and try to give a little space when it comes to some of the relatively harmless decisions they make about their clothing and grooming habits.

- ✔ **Keep the lines of communication open:** Take the time to pay undivided attention to your kid's concerns. It's important to keep the lines of communication open, even if your child seems to want to withdraw.

- ✔ **Don't lecture on the subject:** Try to avoid telling your child what to do. Instead, pay careful attention and you may discover more about the issues causing his problems.

Detecting depression in teens

It is common for adolescents — or anybody for that matter — to occasionally feel unhappy. However, when the unhappiness lasts for more than two weeks, and the teen experiences other symptoms, then he may be suffering from depression. Determining if a teenager is depressed can be a very tricky undertaking. Dramatic physical and mental changes seem to take place almost overnight and it sometimes seems hard to tell the "normal" from the "abnormal."

Depression is a more commonly recognized condition in adolescents than it had been in the past. Parents should look for common signs of depression in adolescents and they should be dealt with in a serious manner and not just passed off as "growing pains" or the normal consequence of adolescence. If you observe some of the signs or behaviors listed in the following bulleted list, they may be indicators of depression. They're not always diagnostic of teen depression; however, they may indicate other psychological, social, family, or school problems. Among these are:

✔ Sadness, anxiety, or a feeling of hopelessness

✔ A sudden drop in grades

✔ Loss of interest in food or compulsive overeating that results in rapid weight loss or gain

✔ Staying awake at night and sleeping during the day

✔ Withdrawal from friends

✔ Unusual irritability, rebellious behavior, or cutting school

✔ Physical complaints, such as headaches, stomachaches, low back pain, or excessive fatigue

✔ Use of alcohol or drugs

✔ Promiscuous sexual activity

✔ A preoccupation with death and dying

Don't be afraid to talk to your child about feelings. If you sense a change or that something is seriously troubling your child, you may be right. You can even ask about suicidal thoughts. You won't increase the possibility of suicidal behavior by asking if someone has thought about it. Asking such a question does not "put thoughts into their heads" but rather is more likely to identify if they may be at risk.

If you or your loved one is finding it extremely difficult or impossible to handle the emotional aspects of acne, get help. And, if you don't feel that you can communicate effectively with your adolescent, get help. Talk to your pediatrician or primary care practitioner or ask for a referral for counseling. Strong suicidal thoughts are an emergency and call for immediate action. Don't go it alone.

Accutane and depression: Is there a link?

For several years, there has been debate over whether Accutane (isotretinoin), a drug prescribed for serious cases of acne, could be causing depression that results in suicide in teenagers taking this powerful medication. Turn to Chapter 13, where I take on this controversial debate about this drug and its generic formulations.

Lots of kids with acne who have *never* taken Accutane are depressed. Moreover, since Accutane was introduced in 1982, it's likely that depression during this time has decreased in those who sorely needed the drug and were successfully treated with it.

Recognizing acne as a feature of emotional disorders

When self-esteem and self-image become an overwhelming preoccupation in some people, they may show signs and symptoms of types of acne that have severe underlying emotional and psychiatric underpinnings.

✔ **Acne excorieé.** This is a self-inflicted skin condition in which the sufferer has a compulsive, irresistible urge to manipulate their skin and to pick real, as well as imagined, acne lesions. This results in a worsening of acne and sometimes scarring of the face. Also known as *acne excorieé des jeunes filles,* this type of acne is almost invariably seen in young females. *Jeunes filles* means "young girls" in French, but this condition is also seen in adult women (and males aren't immune).

Many of these females deny that they manipulate their skin, but it's rather obvious when you can see scabs that are almost always present on their faces. It's assumed that they have an underlying *obsessive-compulsive disorder,* a type of emotional problem characterized by persistent thoughts and ideas and repetitive behavior.

✔ **Body Dysmorphic Disorder (BDD).** This psychiatric condition is characterized by a fixation and chronic complaining about a nonexistent or minimal cosmetic defect or minor flaw in one's physical appearance. The "flaw" can be wrinkles, large pores, or just a few pimples. The person with BDD exhibits an unreasonable amount of anguish about them. BDD occurs equally in males and females.

BDD often results in significant suffering and social difficulties. Individuals with BDD have variable degrees of awareness concerning the psychiatric nature of the illness. Many people continue to agonize about an imagined defect although they're aware that their concerns are excessive, while other folks have no insight into their unusual preoccupation with their appearance. Some people with BDD frequently develop major depressive episodes and are at risk for suicide.

Treating acne excoriée and BDD is a major challenge. Certain medications and cognitive-behavior therapies can complement each other and be helpful for some people. *Cognitive-behavior therapy* involves discovering, challenging, and changing the underlying negative thoughts and beliefs that the people with these conditions repetitively dwell upon.

In addition to these treatments, family education and counseling, to help family members understand what's going on and how to help the sufferer, and group therapy may be of benefit. Unfortunately, individuals with acne excoriée and BDD often refuse psychiatric referral because of their poor insight into the underlying psychiatric illness.

Thinking about Therapy

Your dermatologist, internist, pediatrician, school nurse, school counselor, or other healthcare provider may be able to steer you in the right direction and find someone who can help you or your child contend with some of these emotional issues while they work on the physical ones.

The good news is that the vast majority of people suffering from depression can be treated successfully. Speak to your doctor about the way you feel and ask her to treat you or your child or to make a referral to a psychologist or psychiatrist.

Ideally, you or your child's primary care provider or psychotherapist should maintain a close relationship with your dermatologist so that they can discuss treatment and any changes in medications, and so on.

There are many types of psychotherapy and psychotherapists. You can choose from:

- ✔ **Psychiatrists:** They are medical doctors and are able to prescribe prescription medications, if required.

- ✔ **Clinical psychologists:** They usually have a master's or doctoral degree in psychology.

- ✔ **Psychiatric social workers:** To become qualified as a social worker that provides psychotherapy, a person must have earned a minimum of a master's degree in clinical social work.

- ✔ **Counselors:** Generally, they may have only a bachelor's degree in education, psychology, or theology.

Some dermatologists, albeit few and far between, are capable of handling both the physical and emotional consequences of acne. Several of my colleagues have been trained as dermatologists as well as psychologists and psychiatrists. If you're fortunate to have access to any of these specialists, go for it!

Avoid quick fixes promised by audio and videotapes or books. You can't find true "quickie cures" for acne or for its emotional components. Both sets of symptoms require time and patience.

Chapter 18

Reining in Rosacea and Other Acne Look-Alikes

A 33-year-old woman entered my office in tears. Her face and nose were red as a beet and she had red pimples on her chin, cheeks, and forehead. "Not only do I look horrible, but when people look at me, I'm sure they think I'm an alcoholic! I've always had perfectly clear skin; I didn't even have a pimple when I was a teenager," she said. "I can't cover it with makeup and I hate to leave the house!"

She said that her problem started about a year before when she first noticed a tendency to flush and blush more readily than usual. In time, her face became persistently red, and then she started getting pimples and visible blood vessels on her cheeks, forehead, chin, and nose. It was an easy diagnosis for me to make: She had all the signs and symptoms of rosacea!

Rosacea (pronounced rose-*ay*-shah) is a common skin disorder that is frequently mistaken for acne. In fact, as recently as 20 years ago, rosacea was referred to as *acne rosacea*. In this chapter, I give you details about what rosacea is, how to treat it, and how to cover it up while you're waiting for it to clear up. I also help you figure out what conditions aren't rosacea even though they may look like it.

Rosacea 101

It's easy to understand why rosacea was called "acne rosacea" for so many years, because rosacea and acne look so much alike. They both have red papules and pustules and, of course, appear on the face.

Rosacea occurs at a time in adults' lives when they don't expect to have to deal with pimples and the flushing and blushing reactions of the condition. For adults in the prime years of their careers, the psychological effects of rosacea can pose problems. (In Chapter 17, I cover the emotional tolls that affect some people who have acne. It seems that rosacea can have a similar psychological impact on people's lives.)

However, just as with teenage acne, it's important as an adult to continually remind yourself of an important fact: Your rosacea is treatable and your emotional well-being will improve following successful treatment. Later in this chapter, I show you the many methods that are available to treat your rosacea.

Describing those affected

Anyone can develop rosacea. However, people from certain ethnic backgrounds are most likely to get it. If you have fair skin and have ancestors hailing from Great Britain (including Ireland, Scotland, and Wales), Germany, and Scandinavia, or certain areas of Eastern Europe, you have the greatest tendency to have rosacea. The condition is rare in Hispanic, African, and African-American populations along with other dark-skinned people.

Women are affected with rosacea two to three times more often than men. And if you're between 30 and 50 years of age, have fair skin, blonde hair, blue eyes, and have the proper hereditary pedigree, you're in the higher-risk group to develop rosacea. (For more on the causes, see the "So, what causes rosacea?" section, later in the chapter.)

Heredity plays the major role in whether you develop rosacea. If you flush or blush easily and have a family member who has been diagnosed with rosacea, you're at greater risk for getting it.

Reporting the signs and symptoms

Rosacea may first appear as *erythema* (redness of the skin) on your cheeks and forehead that later spreads to your nose and chin.

These areas comprise the central one-third of the face. Very often, people who have rosacea describe how they're inclined to flush and blush easily. This condition occurs whenever a blood vessel *dilates* (widens). When the blood vessel dilates, it then contains a greater volume of blood, which produces redness. When a person develops *persistent erythema* (abnormal redness), the condition usually doesn't go away on its own.

As rosacea progresses, three main lesions arise against the background of erythema — two of which are very similar and generally indistinguishable in appearance from the acne lesions I cover in Chapter 3. However, they look different when examined by a microscope. The three main rosacea lesions are

- **Telangiectasias:** Many people refer to telangiectasias (tell-*an*-jek-*tay*-shas) as broken blood vessels, but there's nothing broken about them. They're actually enlarged blood vessels that look like thin red lines on the face, especially on the cheeks. Sometimes the tiny vessels look like the shape of a spider (*spider telangiectasias*). Telangiectasias can be more than "tiny" in some folks. I explain their treatment in the "Managing the Redness" section, at the end of this chapter.

- **Papules:** These tiny red pimples appear as small, firm, red bumps. Papules are the primary inflammatory lesion in rosacea.

- **Pustules:** These are mature papules that contain visible pus. Pustules are generally found in the company of papules. Papules are also inflammatory lesions, but they're not as common as papules in rosacea.

The papules and pustules tend to come and go, but the telangiectasias stay put. Rosacea lesions tend to be spread symmetrically on the face, but on occasion, the lesions may occur on only one side of a person's face. Take a look at the color section in this book to see what typical rosacea looks like.

Rosacea is typically a longer lasting condition than acne vulgaris (teenage acne) and adult-onset acne (I talk about them in Chapter 4 and 5, respectively) because it can go on and on through one's adult life. Rosacea also requires somewhat different therapy than acne. The good news is that rosacea is generally easier to treat than are most cases of acne, and I detail the many effective treatments that are available later in this chapter.

Addressing additional signs and symptoms

Lesions of rosacea are most typically seen on the central third of the face — the forehead, the lower half of the nose, the cheeks, and chin. However, additional rosacea-related problems involving the eyes and nose may occur.

The eyes have it: Ocular rosacea

Like acne, for the most part, rosacea is a cosmetic problem; however, some people who have rosacea may also have eye involvement, known as *ocular rosacea*. Ocular rosacea is most frequently noted when rosacea of the skin is also present; however, eye symptoms may precede the skin manifestations in up to 20 percent of people.

The eyes of patients with ocular rosacea may:

- ✔ Feel irritated and gritty as if there is something in their eyes
- ✔ Tend to look bloodshot
- ✔ Become overly sensitive to light

If you have these symptoms, you should consult your doctor or an *ophthalmologist* (a medical doctor that specializes in eye disorders) to establish the correct diagnosis and to get appropriate therapy. Sometimes, the use of prescription eye drops will help improve ocular rosacea, and sometimes, oral antibiotics are prescribed to treat it.

Many people who have ocular rosacea mistakenly think they have pollen or other airborne allergies.

The nose has it: Rhinophyma

Rhinophyma (*rye-no-fie-*mah) can be an unsightly manifestation of rosacea (see the color section of this book). Rhinophyma occurs when oil glands enlarge and a bulbous, red nose develops. This condition usually occurs in men over 40. It consists of knobby bumps that tend, over time, to get larger and swollen. It is quite uncommon and is rarely seen in women. In jolly old England, this type of nose was referred to as "drinker's nose" or "grog blossoms."

The usual treatments that are described in this chapter to treat rosacea don't work very well on rhinophyma, but it can be successfully treated with surgery and special lasers that I tell you about in the "Going the surgical route for rhinophyma," section, later in this chapter.

Comparing the appearance to acne

Despite their similarities, rosacea is different from acne vulgaris and adult-onset acne in many ways. Rosacea

- ✔ **Lacks the mature comedones (blackheads and whiteheads) seen in acne vulgaris.** Lesions are generally small, pimple-like bumps and telangiectasias (tiny, visible blood vessels in the surface of the skin); in contrast, acne lesions are varied and may include comedones, as well as small or large nodules and cysts, but no telangiectasias.

- ✔ **Doesn't seem to have a hormonal connection.** The micro-comedo, the primary lesion of acne vulgaris that I describe in Chapter 3, arises in response to hormonal (androgenic) stimulation, whereas rosacea seems to arise "out of the blue" — or should I say "red" — and doesn't appear to have any relationship to androgenic hormones. Also, lesions don't appear to fluctuate with a woman's menstrual cycle.

- ✔ **Usually makes its debut well after the acne-prone years.** Acne vulgaris is especially common during adolescence.

- ✔ **Occurs primarily on the central face.** Adult-onset acne tends to occur on the lower part of the face and acne vulgaris generally has a much wider distribution such as on the chest and back.

- ✔ **Is associated with facial redness and flushing.** Blushing and flushing reactions aren't associated with acne vulgaris or adult-onset acne.

- ✔ **Is generally non-scarring, unless acne vulgaris is also present.** Fortunately, the inflammatory lesions of rosacea tend to heal without forming the types of scars that can result from inflammatory acne lesions.

Determining whether it's just rosy cheeks

If you believe the ads, we have 15 million and counting rosacea sufferers in the United States alone! You may fit the profile — fair-skinned, Celtic ancestry, and all that. You may show varying degrees of facial redness and blushing and flushing, but that doesn't mean you have rosacea. So don't be in a rush to volunteer as a poster child for rosacea.

Rosacea is a condition that is regularly overdiagnosed by healthcare providers. What's more, many people come into my office after having diagnosed *themselves* as having rosacea. Some of these self-diagnosers reach their conclusion after seeing ask-your-doctor television advertisements that introduce them to the condition.

In many instances, rosacea can be hard to distinguish from weathered, sun-damaged skin that's seen in many fair-skinned farmers, gardeners, sailors, or other folks that worked or spent long periods of their lives outdoors. Such long-term sun exposure can lead to persistent red faces and tiny broken blood vessels that sometimes look quite a bit like rosacea.

Then, some people are blushers who don't have rosacea at all. In fact, if you carefully evaluate the location of redness on some of their faces, you discover that the redness seems to occur in different places than where it's commonly seen in rosacea. Their symptoms tend to appear on the sides of the cheeks, the front and side of the neck, and the ears, as opposed to the central area of the face.

Moreover, a red face can be due to a variety of skin disorders such as *photo dermatitis* (an abnormal reaction to light exposure) and *seborrheic dermatitis* (a red, scaly rash that can be on the face), and sometimes it can be associated with certain underlying diseases such as systemic lupus erythematosus, as well as rarer disorders (such as carcinoid syndrome and systemic mastocytosis). The so-called hot flashes of menopause, medication reactions, and allergy to cosmetics can also be confused with rosacea.

And sometimes, what has been called "rosacea" on your face — is simply rosy cheeks! You're just stuck with a healthy looking facial glow. Traditionally, folks like you didn't receive a medical diagnosis but were described as having a "peaches and cream" complexion.

If rosy cheeks and telangiectasias are your only complaint, you shouldn't be labeled with the diagnosis of rosacea until other signs or symptoms develop such as those I describe in this chapter. Now, if you've decided by now that you don't think you have rosacea, please give this book to a friend or family member who has acne or rosacea.

So, what causes rosacea?

Although the precise cause of rosacea remains a mystery, researchers believe that heredity plays a role in the process (as I cover in the "Describing those affected" section, earlier in the chapter). As to the physical causes of the condition, there are many theories, but none of them have been proven. The various theories about the actual causes include:

- ✔ **Blood vessels:** Some investigators believe that there is a natural chemical in the body that has a potent effect on blood vessels and that causes them to swell in people who have rosacea. The result, these scientists believe, is the flushing and redness characteristic of rosacea.

- ✔ **Bacteria:** A bacterium called *Helicobacter pylori,* which causes intestinal peptic ulcers, was thought to be a cause of rosacea, but that theory has apparently been put to rest. *P. acnes,* our little bacterial friend that's been associated with acne, is also believed by some investigators to play a role in rosacea. I introduce you to *P. acnes* in Chapter 3.

- ✔ **Mites:** A mite called *Demodex folliculorum,* which lives in hair follicles, is thought by some scientists to be the cause of rosacea. The belief is that the mites clog oil glands, which leads to the inflammation seen in rosacea. These mites reside in almost everyone's skin and, like *P. acnes,* may just be innocent bystanders.

Examining Irritants and Rosacea-Prone Skin

If you have rosacea, you may also have skin that is unusually vulnerable to chemical and physical irritants. Skin-care should be kept simple so as to avoid the triggers that can worsen the condition.

Handling your skin with care!

Avoid overzealous washing of your face. Be gentle with your skin. You should wash your face with lukewarm water and a mild, non-irritating soap, by using your fingertips to apply the soap gently. Check out my complete instructions for proper face washing in Chapter 2.

Cosmetics can irritate rosacea; so don't use skin-care products with harsh ingredients. Before using any skin-care products, carefully read the labels. Go for the fragrance-free products that are gentle and have the fewest ingredients.

Celebrity rosacea

If you have rosacea, then you have something in common with the following prestigious group of people:

✔ **Rembrandt van Rijn:** The great Dutch painter, who created a series of self-portraits as he aged, was known for his honest rendering of his facial features. A recent medical journal studied his self-portraits and concluded that he may have had rosacea. A blotch under the right eye looks like spider's legs and resembles a telangiectasia lesion. The bulbous nose with coarse skin suggests that he had *rhinophyma.*

✔ **J. P. Morgan:** The financier, who had a humungous rhinophyma, offered $100,000 to anyone discovering its cause. As far as I know, no one has received payment so far (he died in 1913).

✔ **W. C. Fields:** The sharp-tongued comedian is also among those said to have had rosacea. Just like J. P. Morgan, his trademark bulbous nose resulted from it. Everyone thinks his nose looked that way because of his drinking, when in fact it was due to rosacea. However, there's little doubt that alcohol flushed his face and worsened his rosacea.

✔ **Bill Clinton:** The former United States president reportedly flushes and has a swollen red nose and red bumps on his chin and on his right cheek. These are all symptoms of a moderate case of rosacea.

✔ **Princess Diana:** She reportedly had a mild case of rosacea that she was able to hide under makeup.

The following ingredients seem to cause the most irritation:

- ✔ Alcohol
- ✔ Witch hazel
- ✔ Menthol
- ✔ Peppermint
- ✔ Eucalyptus oil
- ✔ Clove oil
- ✔ Salicylic acid

In choosing cosmetics, also keep the following points in mind:

- ✔ Select cosmetics that are water soluble, so that they require no strong solvents to remove them.
- ✔ Avoid astringents and exfoliating agents.

- ✔ Look for water-based moisturizers.

- ✔ Look for makeup and moisturizers with a sunscreen already added.

- ✔ Opt for powdered blushes because, unlike creams, they're unlikely to contain emulsifiers that can irritate rosacea.

- ✔ Discard your old, spoiled cosmetic products.

As for sunscreens, try to stick with the ones that contain zinc oxide or titanium dioxide, the barrier sunscreens, especially if other sunscreens irritate or worsen your rosacea (see the section "Making it worse — fact and fiction," where I describe them).

For men who have difficulty shaving around the bumps of rosacea, try using an electric razor rather than a blade to reduce abrasion. Also avoid using after-shave lotions, especially those containing alcohol. I describe shaving bumps and shaving techniques in Chapter 19.

Making it worse — fact and fiction

In the following sections, I investigate some things that may make rosacea worse. I start off with the stuff that most dermatologists tend to agree about and then I discuss more questionable items.

Avoiding the triggers

If you do have rosacea, you can take steps to avoid making your condition worse. Here are common triggers you should avoid:

- ✔ **Sun exposure:** You should avoid excessive sun exposure, particularly during the midday. Steer clear of UV tanning lamps and beds.

  Sun protection is extremely important for anyone with rosacea. Sunscreens and sun blockers should be used regularly and liberally to protect the face. Use sunscreens with an SPF factor of 15 or higher. If chemical sunscreens cause stinging, irritation, or worsening of your rosacea, switch to physical barrier sun blocks, which contain titanium dioxide or zinc oxide.

- ✔ **Medications:** The use of *topical corticosteroids* (anti-inflammatory medications used for many skin conditions) can cause a condition similar to rosacea known as steroid-induced rosacea. I discuss this condition in "Being aware of topical steroid-induced 'rosacea'" later in this chapter.

Booze and bumps?

Many in the medical profession thought that drinking brought on a continual *dilatation* (widening) of facial blood vessels and an increase in blood flow to the skin. The increase in blood flow was thought to lead to the thready little broken blood vessels on the cheeks, the reddened "drinker's nose," and ultimately to the skin condition known as rosacea. We now know that the booze doesn't cause the bumps!

✔ **Excess alcohol ingestion:** First of all, let's get one thing straight: Rosacea is *not* caused by drinking excessive amounts of alcohol! That's a serious misconception that's been around for ages and should be put to rest! Traditionally, most doctors believed that many, if not most, cases of rosacea were caused by excessive alcohol intake. It's an unfortunate belief that still persists among the general public.

Hold on, not so fast! That doesn't mean that you should go dashing to your liquor cabinet for that single malt or to your fridge to reach for that six-pack! Though drinking habits have nothing to do with *causing* rosacea, it is accepted that the blushing and flushing of rosacea may flare up when some people drink alcohol — especially red wine. It's questionable, however, that the drinking of alcoholic beverages causes a long-term worsening of the condition.

Questioning the doubtful candidates

There is no convincing evidence as to whether the following factors — I call them my "doubtful candidates" — have any *long-term* harmful effects on rosacea. But, they do increase the redness of the face temporarily:

✔ **Spicy foods, smoking, and caffeine:** These items have been known to cause facial reddening in some people who have rosacea.

✔ **Cooking over a hot stove or oven:** Overheating or flushing from high temperatures in the kitchen has been reported as a reason for rosacea to flare up.

✔ **Emotional stress:** Just cry or get angry and your face may turn red. Just as in the case of acne, some dermatologists think stress worsens rosacea. They believe that at times of stress, the body releases lots more glucocorticoids (the body's natural steroids), which can worsen rosacea.

✔ **Physical exertion:** Exercise if you're fair and you'll flush. Yes, some folks who have rosacea feel that exercise makes it worse.

The extensive trigger list: Mission impossible

It seems that *anything* and *everything* has been reported to cause rosacea flare-ups! The following list obtained from questionnaires sent to rosacea sufferers will prove the point. It reads like everything that's good, nutritious, or fun to do in the entire world:

Foods: Liver, citrus fruits, tomatoes, chocolate, soy sauce, vinegar, and some cheeses. Also foods high in niacin (a B vitamin) or histamine.

Climate: Extremely hot or cold temperatures and the wind. These conditions increase blood flow and cause the small blood vessels in the face to widen.

Other tripwires: Menopause, stress, hot water, fragrant skin-care products, and certain perfumes have also been implicated in the survey. Also included are certain medical conditions such as high blood pressure, fever, and colds.

So why don't you become a hermit and move into a dark cave? Just kidding! If you notice that something does affect your rosacea on a consistent basis, discuss it with your doctor, otherwise, I recommend that you continue to go outside, eat, and live your life.

Of course, a hot shower also makes your face turn red! You obviously can't avoid some of the things on the list — and in some cases, doing so would be bad for your health and turn you into a "couch potato." However, because I'm a doctor, I must recommend changing important lifestyle habits such as giving up smoking and cutting back on your caffeine intake. Remember, you'll receive many more health benefits besides possible improvement in your rosacea by doing so.

Treating Rosacea

Most mild cases of rosacea can be treated and controlled with topical agents alone. (*Topical* refers to a product that is used on the skin, such as a cream, ointment, lotion, foam, gel, or a cleanser.) However, if topical treatment isn't doing the job, an oral antibiotic is generally prescribed *(systemic therapy)*. Compared with topical therapy, systemic therapy has a more rapid onset of action.

If possible, your doctor will try to control your rosacea on a long-term basis with topical therapy alone. Oral antibiotics (check out the next section) are reserved for initial control of rosacea and for breakthrough flare-ups.

In my practice, I start patients off with both an oral antibiotic such as a tetracycline (see the section on tetracycline later in this chapter) as well as a topical medication such as a metronidazole (see the section on metronidazole later in this chapter). That's because it may take a topical agent six to eight weeks for an acceptable therapeutic response, whereas oral antibiotics start working in a week or two. As my patient improves, the dosage of the oral antibiotic is gradually reduced and then stopped.

The goal of combination topical/oral treatment is to produce clearing of rosacea and to maintain it, if possible, with topical therapy alone.

The topical and oral drugs that I describe in the following sections have an anti-inflammatory action that helps to clear up the papules and pustules of mild to moderate rosacea. However, these drugs aren't effective in clearing up the flushing, blushing, and persistent redness (telangiectasias) of rosacea. I talk about treatment of these signs and symptoms of rosacea in the section "Managing the Redness," later in this chapter. All of the medications that I mention in that section require a prescription.

Taking a look at the topicals

Some of the topical medications that are used to treat acne can be used very effectively on rosacea; however, some precautions must be taken because many people who have rosacea also have very sensitive skin. Consequently, standard acne medications such as topical retinoids and benzoyl peroxide can be drying and irritating. Retinoids may sometimes even sensitize the skin to the sun and worsen rosacea. Despite my reservations, if your skin tolerates these products without any irritation, there's no reason not to use them, particularly if they work. I talk about all of these agents in Chapter 9.

Just as we use topical agents in combination with each other (or in combination with oral agents) in the treatment of acne, this approach has become popular for managing rosacea too. On the subject of combining topical treatments, Noritate cream applied at night and a sodium sulfacetamide/sulfur product such as Ovace, Klaron, or Avar applied in the morning appear to work better than when each of these agents is used alone.

In this section, though, I discuss topical medications that are used to treat rosacea. You may recognize a few familiar friends such as azelaic acid and sodium sulfacetamide and sulfur that I discuss in Chapter 9 that are sometimes used to treat acne. Doctors and researchers aren't sure exactly how the following medications work in the treatment of rosacea, but it does appear that it's mostly due to an anti-inflammatory effect.

Each of these products is considered to be as effective as the others in the treatment of rosacea.

Metronidazole

Metronidazole is the most frequently prescribed first-line topical therapy for rosacea. Irritation and burning are uncommon from these topical medications, especially when the creams are used. They're generally prescribed as one of the following:

- **MetroCream, MetroGel, and MetroLotion:** Commonly referred to as the Metros, all of these products contain 0.75 percent metronidazole. The Metros are applied twice a day to clean dry skin on the rosacea-prone areas.

  The latest Metro is the higher strength 1 percent MetroGel that's applied once daily. Besides having a higher concentration of metronidazole, it's a water-based formulation that contains niacinamide, which is thought to have anti-inflammatory effects.

- **Noritate cream:** This product is similar to MetroCream, but with 1 percent metronidazole, it's 25 percent stronger than the Metros. Noritate ("no irritate," get it?) is used only once a day, a routine that helps patients use it regularly.

Azelaic acid

This gel is used to improve the inflammatory pimples of mild to moderate rosacea. Finacea and Skinoren (in Europe) are the brand names available. Finacea is available in a 15 percent azelaic acid gel. They're applied twice a day to clean dry skin. Some patients report temporary burning or stinging with this treatment.

If you have a dark complexion, your doctor should monitor you for signs of skin lightening.

Sodium sulfacetamide and sulfur

Medications containing sodium sulfacetamide and sulfur are also effective for rosacea. Brand names include Klaron, Plexion, Rosula, Rosac, Rosanil, Novacet, and Ovace, to name a few.

Sodium sulfacetamide and sulfur products are available as lotions, creams, and washes. Some of these products contain a *humectant* (a substance that promotes retention of moisture) and can be used in rosacea patients who have dry, sensitive skin.

These products are generally applied twice a day to clean dry skin. Itching, stinging, and irritation may occur with these preparations.

Treating rosacea by mouth

The same systemic oral antibiotics used to treat acne that I discuss in Chapter 10 also calm the papules and pustules of your rosacea. Here, I provide you with the rosacea-specific information and tips associated with these drugs. For complete information, including how to take the medication and potential side effects, please see Chapter 10. Of course, your doctor always has the last word on these prescription drugs.

Whenever any systemic drugs are taken, the potential dangers — including side effects, drug allergy, drug intolerance, drug inter-actions, and fetal exposure in women who are, or may become pregnant — must be carefully considered.

Tetracycline and tetracycline derivatives, such as minocycline and doxycycline, are the first-line oral drugs of choice in the management of moderate to severe rosacea. The tetracyclines are antibiotics. They have antibacterial properties and many uses besides treating rosacea, but as far as rosacea is concerned, this antibiotic has a powerful anti-inflammatory action that helps to clear up the papules and pustules.

With the tetracyclines, improvement of rosacea is usually noticeable in a matter of a week or two. The papules and pustules begin to flatten and disappear and new ones stop popping up. Tetracyclines are then tapered when this improvement becomes persistent (usually after three to four weeks). Minocycline is probably the most effective oral medication to treat rosacea. It's also the most expensive.

None of the tetracyclines should be used if you're pregnant or breastfeeding.

Other oral medications that may be prescribed include:

- **Other antibiotics:** A variety of other oral antibiotics (such as erythromycin, azithromycin, clarithromycin, and amoxicillin) have been used to treat rosacea successfully. Typically they're prescribed as second-line alternatives when a tetracycline fails or isn't tolerated.

- **Oral metronidazole:** This drug's brand name is Flagyl, and it may be used when antibiotics aren't working.

✔ **Trimethoprim sulfasoxazole (TMZ):** Trimethoprim sulfasoxazole is reserved for unusually stubborn cases of severe rosacea that don't respond to any of the other antibiotics listed.

Rarely, TMZ has been associated with severe side effects and may precipitate severe allergic reactions.

Although isotretinoin, better known as Accutane, is extremely effective in the treatment of severe acne, it hasn't been very useful in rosacea. It may clear rosacea, but the improvement is often temporary and the rosacea tends to rebound. In other words, the risks — which are plentiful — are probably not worth the benefits in the treatment of rosacea! Isotretinoin (Accutane) has many potential side effects and I review the ups and downs of this powerful drug in Chapter 13. While isotretinoin (Accutane) hasn't been proven to be very helpful for severe inflammatory rosacea, there have been instances where the drug has demonstrated a reduction of some of the volume of rhinophyma lesions. I talk about the treatment of rhinophyma later in the chapter.

Because rosacea doesn't seem to have a relationship to hormonal fluctuations, the use of hormonal therapy that I mention in Chapter 11 for the treatment of acne has no place in the treatment of rosacea.

Check out Chapter 15 where I delve into old and new alternative and complementary methods to treat acne and rosacea. Herbs reported to help clear rosacea include neem, cat's claw, tea tree, ginger, and lavender. There's no scientific evidence to back up these claims, however.

Managing the Redness

While you're waiting for the medicine to work to relieve you of those bumpy papules and pustules, why not try to conceal the redness? The next section gives you a few helpful pointers, and later in this chapter, I suggest some more permanent ways to get rid of the red.

Covering up with camouflage

Because treatment isn't enough to handle the redness, you may want to consider strategic camouflage techniques.

Green-tinted foundations can hide the red. Green neutralizes red. It's that simple. That explains why your normal shade of beige or other neutral skin tone foundation doesn't quite conceal the redness that peeks out from underneath. Cosmetic foundations that have a green tint are included in the products made by companies such as Este Lauder, Clinique, and Prescriptives.

Other nonprescription products that may be used to cover up the redness are Dermablend and Covermark. They can be matched to your normal skin color. These products can be found in makeup counters in some department stores and also can be obtained online at www.dermablend.com and www.covermark.com.

The prescription cover-up products, Avar (tinted green) and Sulfacet-R, both are tinted and thus offer ways to hide the red. Sulfacet-R is also available in a tint-free preparation and is particularly useful for oily skin. These products can serve as a cosmetic cover-up to hide the "broken" blood vessels and redness of rosacea. Sulfacet-R comes with a color blender so that you can match your skin tones. Both of these are types of sodium sulfacetamide, which I discuss in the section of the same name earlier in the chapter.

Buzzing the telangiectasias away

Your dermatologist can treat your telangiectasias by *electrocautery* — destroying them with a tiny electric needle using extremely low voltage electricity. The needle zaps along the length of the blood vessel and destroys it. Simple electrocautery tends to be sufficient for most small telangiectasias; it is relatively painless, and is the most cost effective approach to get rid of telangiectasias.

For the larger variety of telangiectasia, lasers such as I describe in the next section may be the treatment of choice.

Your insurance will probably not cover these procedures, because they're considered to be cosmetic in nature.

Getting the red out: Light-based therapies

Topical and oral therapies don't treat the telangiectasias or the larger, persistent erythematous (red) areas of rosacea. Special lasers known as *vascular lasers* and *intense pulsed light* (IPL) therapy are now being used by dermatologists and plastic surgeons to "erase" this red background away.

Light-based therapies use various wavelengths of light to penetrate the skin and target the blood vessels on the face and cause the vessels to heat up and collapse.

These light treatments haven't proven to be effective for flushing and blushing reactions, nor do they seem to be superior to oral antibiotics in treating the inflammatory component of rosacea. All of this is still in an early, investigational phase. The treatments are very expensive and generally not covered by health insurance plans. I shed more light on lasers and IPL in Chapter 14.

Going the surgical route for rhinophyma

Recontouring procedures with a scalpel or a carbon dioxide laser have been used successfully to "sculpt" the excess nose tissue of rhinophyma back down to a more normal shape and appearance. This may also be accomplished by *electrocautery,* a process of destroying tissue by using a small electric probe to *cauterize* (burn or destroy) unwanted tissue, or by dermabrasion. Results can last for many years and sometimes may be permanent. I explain dermabrasion, carbon dioxide lasers, and other surgical measures in Chapter 16.

Dermatologic or plastic surgeons perform these procedures. Health insurance plans are generally very reluctant about covering such treatments, which they consider to be "cosmetic" in nature.

Identifying Rosacea Look-Alikes

The conditions that I mention in the following sections are really impossible to differentiate from rosacea except in three respects: they're usually easy to treat, they generally disappear on their own (self-limiting), and they tend to show up in different areas of the face than does rosacea.

Recognizing perioral dermatitis

Also known as *periorificial dermatitis,* this condition is a rosacea-like skin eruption seen almost exclusively in women. Like rosacea, nobody knows its cause. Fluoridated toothpastes and bacteria have occasionally been implicated, but without any consistent evidence.

Perioral dermatitis occurs in a characteristic circular pattern around the mouth, chin, and lower cheek in women between the ages of 15 and 40 years. Less commonly, it can occur in young children. The lesions look just like those of rosacea or acne and consist of papules and pustules, except there are no telangiectasias. The papules and pustules tend to be very small, and sometimes whitish scales can be associated with it. Take a look at the color section of this book to see what this condition looks like.

The biggest difference between rosacea, acne, and perioral dermatitis is that the latter often clears up permanently after treatment.

Perioral dermatitis is usually found clustered around the mouth, but it may appear around the eyes and nose.

Treatment is similar to that of rosacea. The use of topical MetroGel or Noritate cream or topical antibiotics such as Cleocin T or Emgel can help to clear up this condition, especially for mild cases. An oral antibiotic such as one of the tetracyclines or erythromycin is used if topical treatment fails.

Being aware of topical steroid-induced "rosacea"

Also called *steroid rosacea,* this type of "rosacea" isn't really rosacea, and I *can* tell you the cause of this condition — the inappropriate use of topical steroids (cortisone) on the face. The steroid creams are often prescribed for other skin conditions such as eczema or psoriasis and then overused by the unsuspecting person who continues to apply them. The condition typically worsens when the topical steroids are discontinued (an occurrence known as *rebound rosacea*).

Here's what happens: There is a rapid flare of papules and pustules when the topical steroid is stopped, so the unsuspecting person reapplies the offending medication and the condition improves. When the treatment is stopped again, the lesions appear again and reestablish the vicious cycle. Some of my dermatology colleagues refer to this as *steroid-use dermatitis* (others replace the term "use" with "abuse" or "misuse").

It looks just like ordinary rosacea, but a history of long-term, indiscriminate misuse of potent topical steroids on the face helps to confirm the diagnosis. This condition is treated by *stopping* the topical steroids and by taking a tetracycline derivative for a few weeks or more to get over the hump of the rebound.

Chapter 19

Fighting the Feisty Follicle

*I*t seems like this entire book takes place in, or has to do with, your hair follicles. When a hair follicle becomes inflamed, it may become a papule or a pustule and look just like acne! Yes, there are more "acne pretenders" besides the ones I talk about in Chapter 18. In this chapter, I further explore your hair follicle, a place that can also serve as a location for other pretenders — razor bumps and *keratosis pilaris.*

Reining in Razor Bumps

If you're a guy with curly hair (and much less often a woman), the area under your chin, upper neck, or cheeks can be subject to an uncomfortable cluster of papules and sometimes pustules, which can make shaving very difficult. This condition is known as *pseudofolliculitis barbae* (PFB); more commonly called *razor bumps.* That's right, "pseudo" as in phony. Although no one would argue that your inflamed follicles are fake, your condition isn't actually folliculitis.

The term *folliculitis* simply refers to any inflammation or infection of hair follicles.

Besides being a cosmetic liability, these bumps can really become itchy, painful, and tender. In addition to the papules and pustules, if the condition goes unchecked, the following lesions may ultimately result:

> ✔ **Persistent flesh-colored bumps:** These lesions are actually *hypertrophic scars* that sometimes go on and result in *keloids*. I discuss hypertrophic scars and keloids in Chapter 16.
>
> ✔ **PIP:** Postinflammatory pigmentation, or dark spots, may also become a prominent feature on people with PFB. See Chapter 12 for more information on dealing with PIP.

PFB is a condition that can appear in folks from all ethnic backgrounds. It's extremely common in men of African descent as well as some men of Hispanic origin and non-Hispanic Caucasians with curly hair. And yes, it can also be a plague to some women in these groups.

Examining the causes

People with curly hair have curved hair follicles. Most African-American people have curved hair follicles. The majority of Caucasians and virtually all Asians have straight hair follicles that produce straight hairs, which explains why we see more African-American men with PFB. PFB lesions are seen on the beard area — particularly on the neck and below the jawbone. Take a look at the color section of this book for an up-close view of the condition.

Reentry of a hair missile: Ingrown hairs

Because the hair shafts of people with curly hair are curved, the hairs that emerge from their follicles tend to be tightly coiled. It's true of beard hair as well as other body hair. After shaving, a single curly hair becomes a sharply pointed tip that if aimed toward the body, can grow right back into the skin. Figures 19-1A and 19-1B illustrate the process.

The penetration of sharp hairs causes a misguided reaction by your body's immune system that sees your penetrating hairs as "foreign invaders." Your immune system overreacts by attacking the hair with white blood cells and thus produces inflammatory *papules* and *pustules* that resemble acne.

Parallel hair penetration: Shaving below the surface

When they're shaved too closely, hairs can also grow parallel to the skin and penetrate the side of the follicle. Check out Figures 19-1C and 19-1D. This penetration also causes a reaction of your immune system, producing papules and pustules.

Reemerging hairs: Adding insult to injury

Furthermore, newly erupting hairs from below may pierce and aggravate areas that are already inflamed. Thus, growing hair or hairs that have been plucked may traumatize an existing papule or pustule.

 Try your best not to pluck hairs growing in areas in which you have PFB, because new hairs will again grow from below and penetrate a site that is already inflamed. For tips on how to remove hair without causing further problems, see the section "Dealing with Those Hairs," later in this chapter.

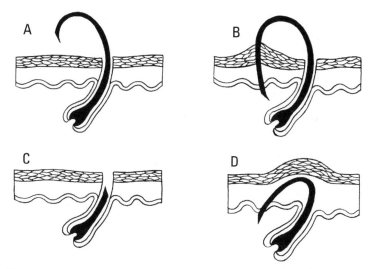

Figure 19-1: When shaved, the curly hair emerging from a curved follicle becomes a sharp tip that curves downward as it grows (A), and reenters the skin (B). When hair is cut too closely (C), it may grow parallel to the skin and penetrate the side of the follicle (D).

Shaving correctly with PFB

If you have PFB, you need to establish proper shaving techniques. Allowing you hairs to grow long enough so they won't grow back into the skin can be helpful, or you might decide to stop shaving permanently! Growing a beard is probably the best way to prevent PFB, though most people don't choose this option.

 If you want to try the stop-shaving approach but you're in the military, law enforcement, or work in a company that requires you to be clean-shaven, ask your healthcare provider to give you a letter that explains your PFB condition and why you should be excused from shaving.

If you intend to keep on shaving, the following sections give you some tips on preventing PFB. The key with all of these techniques is to reduce how close the shave is so that you reduce the chance of ingrown hairs. Hairs cut too short are at risk of curling into the skin while growing and causing more razor bumps.

Whatever method you choose when shaving, be sure to use the sharpest implement.

Razor shaving

Just like washing your face, shaving is a little more complicated than some people think, especially if you're prone to skin problems such as PFB.

You can avoid a close shave by using a guarded razor. Two that I recommend are the PFB Bump Fighter or an Aveeno PFB Bump Fighter Razor. Both of these products should be available at your local drugstore. These razors are covered with a plastic coating that prevents the razor from contacting the skin directly and produces less trauma to the skin.

Here are my tips for shaving in the most pain-free and healthy way:

- Soften your hairs before shaving. Try shaving after you take a warm shower. Steaming helps to soften your beard. Washing your face before shaving removes oil and causes hairs to become more erect, making them easier to cut. Lather the beard area with a non-irritating, lubricating shaving gel such as Aveeno Therapeutic Shave Gel, Edge, or a benzoyl peroxide-containing prescription shaving foam such as BenzaShave.

- Use shaving gels to hydrate your hairs and to provide lubrication between the razor blades and your skin.

- Shave with downward strokes. Go with the grain. Shaving in the same direction that the hair lies (typically down) will result in less pull on the hairs and less tendency to cut them too short. Shaving with the grain will also minimize skin irritation.

- Minimize repeat shaving strokes. Not only is it a waste of time and energy to go over and over the same area, but repeated shaving may result in hairs being cut too short.

- Don't stretch the skin during shaving because this leads to a closer shave and increases the chances of producing ingrown hairs.

- Don't shave on a daily basis if you don't have to.

- Don't use aftershave or cologne on the shaved areas. Instead, after shaving is finished, rinse thoroughly with warm water and apply a mild moisturizing aftershave lotion such as Cetaphil Lotion.

✔ Rinse your razor of all cut hairs at regular intervals. It helps to reduce the drag across the skin. Change your blades at least once a week and more often if skin irritation persists.

✔ Be sure not to use those double, triple, and quadruple razors, which wind up shaving you two, three, and four times! These modern razors are so good at what they do, they shave below the skin surface and only make things worse.

Electric shaving

Using an electric razor with gentle pressure is another method that reduces the closeness of the shave. Just as with a wet razor, an electric razor should be cleaned regularly so that the mechanism doesn't become clogged with hairs.

When using an electric shaver, you want the hairs to be dry and stiff before you begin, so they're easier to cut. So you should *not* start by washing your face or thoroughly wetting the beard with water as you do with a wet shave with a blade.

Instead, you may want to apply a pre-shave lotion designed for electric shavers (such as Lectric Shave). Such products, often alcohol-based, dry up the oils and moisture on your skin and make the whiskers stand straight up.

Try using electric hair clippers that leave the cut hairs long. Aim to have a "five o'clock shadow" immediately after shaving.

Treating razor bumps on your own

The good news about PFB is that it can be treated. You can start by treating it yourself, using the physical method I recommend in the next section. You can also use topical medications that contain benzoyl peroxide (see "Buying benzoyl peroxide," later in this section). If you don't get satisfactory results, contact your dermatologist for help. He can evaluate your condition and help you take the next steps.

Physically stopping PFB

A curled hair can be flipped up before it has a chance to plunge into the skin by using a fine needle or toothpick to gently lift it before reentry.

1. **Inspect your beard to look for potential plunging hairs or for hairs that have already taken the plunge.** Prime candidates include those that are pointing back toward your skin or those that are lying flat.

2. **Use a fine needle or toothpick to lift the hair between the follicle and the tip.**

3. **Gently redirect the sharp pointed end of the hair away from your skin.**

Probing too aggressively with a needle or toothpick can lead to further inflammation.

Buying benzoyl peroxide

Benzoyl peroxide is the most commonly used over-the-counter acne medication, and is also the most effective medication for treating PFB. It comes in varying strengths ranging from 2.5 to 10 percent. There's no proof that anything higher than 2.5 percent works any better than the higher concentration, and the lower concentrations are cheaper and may be less irritating to your skin. Clear By Design, Clearasil, Fostex, Neutrogena, and Noxzema are just a few of the benzoyl peroxide brand names available.

A cream or water-based product may be gentler if your skin is very sensitive; however, alcohol-based products may be more potent if you're able to tolerate them. Experiment with the different products until you find the right one for you.

Here are some application tips:

✔ Apply the benzoyl peroxide sparingly in a very thin layer to the entire PFB-prone areas once or twice a day. You may have to continue applying it for as long as you have the problem, or you can try stopping it for periods of time when the PFB comes under control.

✔ Avoid abrasive, harsh, or drying soaps and cleansers while using benzoyl peroxide.

Be patient, your PFB often responds very slowly to treatment. It may take six to eight weeks before you notice any improvement.

Dryness of the treated area can be expected and is usually mild. You may experience a mild burning sensation or reddening of the skin when you first start to apply benzoyl peroxide. These symptoms usually disappear in two to three weeks. For more information on using benzoyl peroxide, take a look at Chapter 7.

Other OTC products

In addition to benzoyl peroxide, topical fruit acids, such as glycolic acid and salicylic acid, products that contain lactic acid, and mixtures of all three are also advertised as PFB treatments. They're not as effective as benzoyl peroxide, and I only mention glycolic acid here. I provide more details about these acids in Chapter 7.

- **Glycolic acid:** Besides benzoyl peroxide, glycolic acid, which is an *alpha hydroxy acid* (AHA), is the most common ingredient found in over-the-counter PFB products. It's found in many cosmetics and moisturizers. Examples of glycolic acid preparations are Alpha-Hydrox and Neo-Strata. Cleansers containing glycolic acid and other AHAs can be used prior to shaving with a razor and moisturizers that have an AHA in them are recommended after shaving.

- **Hydrocortisone cream:** You can purchase over-the-counter 1 percent hydrocortisone cream, which is topical cortisone for itching or irritation. Apply a small amount once or twice a day for itching or stinging, only if necessary.

Getting professional help

If going it alone isn't working out, you may need to see your dermatologist or healthcare provider about getting a prescription medication for your PFB. (If you don't already have a doctor you trust to help you with this problem, turn to Chapter 8 where I tell you how to go about finding the right doctor for you.)

Combining benzoyl peroxide with topical antibiotics

If over-the-counter isn't working for you, prescription benzoyl peroxide combined with a topical antibiotic such as Benzamycin, Duac, or BenzaClin gel may work very well for you.

To save a little money, you could also talk to your doctor about using a prescription for a generic topical antibiotic such as clindamycin or erythromycin lotion along with an over-the-counter benzoyl peroxide. Use them one on top of the other.

As with applying benzoyl peroxide alone, it may take six to eight weeks for the product to work and the same potential side effects of dryness and irritation may also apply. Benzoyl peroxide also is available as prescription shaving foam known as BenzaShave.

If you have supersensitive skin, prescription Akne-Mycin (erythromycin, 2 percent) ointment may be right for you. It also may take six to eight weeks for it to work. It's less harsh on your skin.

Chapter 9 gives you more information about these drugs, but here are some general tips for using these medications for PFB:

- ✔ Apply medication sparingly in a very thin layer to your PFB-prone areas once or twice a day.

- ✔ If you must shave, apply the medication after you shave. Wait at least 30 minutes to cause the least irritation.

- ✔ Apply a moisturizer over the medicine to help prevent dry skin and other irritation.

Using topical retinoids

As with the treatment of acne, the topical retinoids appear to help reduce the inflammatory lesions of PFB. Topical retinoids can perform a double duty for you. In addition to the beneficial actions of the retinoids in treating some of the inflammatory lesions of PFB, they also lighten PIP (if you have it) as well.

Adaplene (Differin), tazarotene (Tazorac), Avita, and tretinoin (Retin-A) are all prescription retinoids. Check out Chapter 9 for more information about prescription-strength topical acne medication.

Apply topical retinoids in small, thin, pea-sized amounts to the PFB-prone areas. Creams are the least irritating, so you probably should start out with a cream-based retinoid instead of a gel. All retinoids can cause some skin irritation during the first few weeks. You may have some discomfort, such as stinging or burning and, sometimes, mild scaling of your skin. If you have a sensitivity to the retinoid you were prescribed, then use it every other day, or even less frequently, until you get used to it.

Maximal improvement most often occurs within three to four months.

Trying other topical measures

Your dermatologist has a few other topical tools at his disposal. Consider these additions to your topical therapy if you're itching or have dark spots and your doctor feels you need them:

- ✔ A prescription-strength topical cortisone cream may be helpful if you have a great deal of itching or irritation.

- ✔ Glyquin, a combination of glycolic acid and hydroquinone (a bleaching chemical) is a moisturizing cream especially helpful for those with PFB and PIP. Apply it once or twice a day.

Opting for oral antibiotics

When your beard becomes populated with papules and pustules, gets to be super itchy, or your scars seem to be growing, it's time for more aggressive therapy. At times like this, your dermatologist may elect to treat your PFB with oral as well as topical preparations.

Oral antibiotic drugs have an anti-inflammatory action that helps to clear inflammatory lesions (papules and pustules). I discuss the oral antibiotics such as the tetracyclines in detail in Chapter 10.

Injecting the bumps with cortisone

When scars become unsightly or the papules become itchy or painful, a very common method to deal with them is by injecting the lesions with cortisone. The shots are given in addition to oral and topical antibiotics. Intralesional cortisone injections (a relatively painless procedure) can be extremely effective in reducing the inflammation and sometimes the size of inflammatory papules and hypertrophic scars. They also help decrease itching. Check out Chapter 10 to see my explanation for this procedure.

This usually requires repeated treatments because PFB is a chronic problem.

Dealing with Those Hairs

Whether you're a man or a woman, if you discover some dark hairs on your chin, cheeks, or neck, you may find them to be annoying or cosmetically objectionable. If you have PFB, this section offers some ideas to lessen your follicular problems.

Your excess hairs may be due to *hirsutism,* an excess of hair in a masculine pattern seen in women. Hirsutism can be seen in certain cases of hard-to-treat acne. You may also have excessive hair growth on other areas besides your face such as on your chest, nipples, and pubic area (see Chapter 20 where I tell you more about hirsutism). This section provides lots of solutions for this condition as well.

Many methods are available for temporary or permanent hair removal. The following sections go over some different methods.

Removing hairs temporarily

Technically referred to as *epilation,* plucking, tweezing, and waxing are common choices for temporary hair removal. These methods remove the intact hair with its root. Performed by aestheticians or by yourself, these procedures are commonly used and are safe; however, they can sometimes result in irritation and folliculitis. As you may know, your hair will still grow back with these approaches. But contrary to myth, shaving, plucking, and tweezing don't promote heavier hair growth.

Chemical depilatories are another option. Depilatories remove hair from the surface of the skin. They separate the hair from its follicle by destroying the bonds that hold the hairs together. Nair and Neet are commercially available products. For PFB, chemical depilatories such as Magic Shave and Royal Crown Powders are effective in removing and softening hairs. Chemical depilation may be best suited for treatment of large hairy areas in people who are unable to afford more expensive treatments such as electrolysis and laser epilation. The main disadvantages of chemical depilatories are irritation of the skin and the unpleasant odor of the products.

These products dissolve the hairs but can be too strong and cause chemical burns on facial skin.

Sugaring, threading, and camouflaging your hairs

Here are some other ideas for removing and hiding unwanted hairs:

✔ **Sugaring:** This is an ancient method of hair removal, still in use today. "Sugaring" is similar to waxing. Long used in parts of the Middle East, the use of natural sugars is becoming popular in place of waxes. They appear to epilate as effectively as, but less traumatically than, waxing.

The sugar mixture is prepared by heating sugar, lemon juice, and water to form a syrup. A sticky paste is applied to the skin, and a strip of cloth or paper is pressed into the preparation. The strip is then quickly pulled away, taking hairs with it. Many states require a cosmetologist or aesthetician's license to do hair removal like sugaring.

✔ **Threading:** This is a method used in some Middle Eastern countries; cotton threads are used to pull out hairs by their roots. Called *khite* in Arabic, the application involves the use of a long twisted loop of thread rotated rapidly across the skin. By maneuvering the twisted string, hairs are trapped within the tight entwined coils and are pulled or broken off.

✔ **Bleaching:** This is an inexpensive, safe alternative to dark hair removal. It works well when hair growth isn't excessive. Bleaches lighten the color of the hair so that it is less noticeable. Several types of commercial hair bleaching products are available. All contain hydrogen peroxide as their active ingredient.

Until you see how your skin reacts to a chemical depilatory, leave these products on your skin for *less* time than is recommended on the package instructions.

Removing hairs permanently

Techniques of permanent epilation include electrolysis, thermolysis, and laser epilation.

Electrolysis and thermolysis

Hair destruction by electrolysis or thermolysis is performed with a fine, flexible electrical wire (probe) that produces an electrical current after being introduced down the hair shaft. The electricity is delivered to the follicle through the wire, which causes localized damage to the areas that generate hairs.

Thermolysis (diathermy) employs a high-frequency alternating current and is much faster than the traditional electrolysis method, which uses a direct galvanic current. Thermolysis works by causing water molecules in the skin around the probe to vibrate, which creates heat. If enough heat is produced, it can damage the cells that cause hair growth.

Electrolysis and thermolysis are slow processes and require multiple treatments for permanent results.

 Both electrolysis and thermolysis are excellent procedures to accomplish permanent hair removal, however, treatments can be rather uncomfortable and can worsen PFB, create folliculitis, and result in postinflammatory pigmentary (PIP) changes in the skin. These methods are difficult to use on inflammatory lesions.

Make sure to find a competent electrologist. Ask around. One of the best ways to find a good one is to ask friends and family for recommendations. These practitioners can be found in beauty salons, doctor's offices, personal offices, or they may work out of their own homes.

Many states require that electrologists be licensed or certified within the state in order to practice electrolysis. For states that do not regulate electrolysis, look for electrologists who have a certification from an accredited electrology school.

Laser epilation

Lasers can treat larger areas and do it faster than electrolysis and thermolysis. They have skin-cooling mechanisms that minimize skin damage during the procedure. Skin and hair color often determine if a laser should be used. Lasers are most effective on dark hairs on fair-skinned people.

As with electrolysis and thermolysis, multiple treatments are often necessary for long-term hair destruction. Results are inconclusive regarding whether lasers are more effective in permanent hair removal than the more traditional methods such as electrolysis. They're certainly more costly.

In dark-skinned people, the Nd:YAG laser seems to be safe and effective. (In Chapter 14, I talk more about lasers.) This laser is currently the most effective laser for hair removal in dark-skinned individuals who have PFB.

Slowing down the hairs

Vaniqa (eflornithine hydrochloride cream) is a prescription topical cream that works by inhibiting an enzyme required for hair growth. It is indicated for the reduction of unwanted facial hair in women and must be used continuously to be effective. You may notice results after four to eight weeks, but your hair growth will return if you stop using the cream.

Oral treatment with anti-androgens should be considered when hirsutism is associated with an underlying disorder. Androgen inhibition with spironolactone or flutamide is sometimes used when medical reasons are identified as the cause of the hirsutism. All of these drugs must be given continuously because when they're stopped, androgens revert to their former level (see Chapter 20).

Recognizing and Feeling Keratosis Pilaris: "Hair Bumps"

Keratosis pilaris (KP) is a very common skin disorder that tends to run in families. Although the condition isn't serious, it can be frustrating because it's difficult to treat. It begins most often in childhood and often continues into adulthood. KP results from the buildup of *keratin* (coarse proteins in your skin that form your hair and nails) that plugs the openings of hair follicles in the skin. (I talk more about keratin in Chapter 3.)

KP is particularly common in teenagers on the upper arms and it tends to be most obvious when it occurs on the cheeks. Lesions may remain for years but they may gradually diminish or even disappear before age 30. KP can be unsightly, but it is completely harmless. Take a look at the color section of this book for a visual.

Distinguishing KP from acne

KP occurs as small, rough patches — usually on the arms and sometimes on the cheeks. It can also appear on the thighs and buttocks. It causes no pain or itching. It has a sandpaper-like feel to it and looks like gooseflesh. The diagnosis of KP can often be made by simply rubbing the area with your hands. Often, there may be some red papules mixed in with the rough bumps.

I bring the subject of KP up because healthcare providers so often mistake it for acne. The whitish papules tend to look like *closed comedones* (whiteheads) and the red papules tend to resemble the inflammatory lesions of acne, whereas in reality KP is a *disorder of hyperkeratosis* (too much keratin). Check out the color section in this book to see KP up close and personal.

Treating the hair bumps

No cure or very effective treatment is available for KP. However, the good news is that in most people the bumps usually diminish in number with increasing age. Treatment is directed at softening the keratin deposits in the skin and may include medicated creams and lotions that contain either urea, such as Carmol 20, or lactic acid, such as AmLactin Moisturizing Lotion. You can also use petroleum jelly, cold cream, or 2 percent salicylic acid (which removes the top layer of skin) to flatten the pimples. Salicylic acid products and their uses are covered in Chapter 7.

Topical retinoids such as tretinoin, Retin-A Micro, and Differin cream have all been used to treat KP. The results have not been impressive, however.

Chapter 20

Reviewing Endocrine Disorders Associated with Acne

....

....

*B*ecause hormones influence acne, there are instances when acne's presence, coupled with other signs or symptoms, may indicate that something else in your body may be going awry. This is particularly the case if you've found it difficult to get your acne under control. When you've tried many different approaches and your acne remains, your dermatologist or healthcare provider may suspect that you have a hormonal imbalance *(endocrine disorder)*.

In this chapter, I explore some of the more likely endocrine disorders that can produce excessive androgens, as well as those that can manifest with elevated cortisol levels. Both of these hormones can be responsible for producing or aggravating pre-existing acne.

It should be noted that the use of anabolic-androgenic steroids, as performance-enhancing drugs, are known to produce hormonal imbalances and acne in men as well as women. I talk about those hormones in Chapter 6.

When you go for your first visit to have your acne evaluated, you will likely be asked for a complete history about your acne and for other general and specific health information. (For a more complete picture of visiting the dermatologist for the first time, check out Chapter 8.) Many of the questions your doctor asks you are intended to determine if your acne is in any way related to a hormone imbalance or abnormality.

Connecting Androgen Excess and Acne

The most common endocrine-related issue when it comes to acne is *androgen excess*. As I review in Chapter 4, it is thought that males tend to have the more severe cases of acne because they produce much higher levels of androgens than do females; however, far and away, most of the acne-related hormonal problems are seen in women.

Women are the primary sufferers from endocrine imbalances. As in males, androgens also are necessary for the development of acne in females.

If you're female, certain instances call for particular attention to endocrine function and suggest that you're experiencing elevated levels of androgens. The following are possible signs that you should be tested with this in mind:

- ✔ **An evident worsening of your acne or an unresponsiveness to treatment.**

- ✔ **Excessive hair growth on your face and other parts of your body.** Your doctor will ask you if you have excessive hair growth on such areas as your face (particularly the upper lip, chin, cheeks, and temple areas; see the color section of this book); also, you may be asked about hair growth on your chest, nipples, pubic area, upper back, lower back, buttocks, inner thighs, and genitals. If this type of hair growth is present, it is referred to as *hirsutism,* an excess of hair in a masculine pattern.

- ✔ **Thinning of your hair well before menopause.** *Androgenic hair loss* is characterized by decreased hair on the top and the temple areas of the scalp similar to a man's hair loss.

- ✔ **Marked changes in your menstrual cycle.** In your first few years of *menarche* (the beginning of your menstrual periods that usually occur during puberty), it's normal to have irregular menstrual cycles; however, if these irregularities persist, or you go from regular to irregular — or if you never have a period — that may indicate that you have an endocrine abnormality.

- ✔ **Infertility.** An inability to conceive after one year of unprotected intercourse.

✔ **Obesity:** Markedly being overweight or the inability to rid yourself of excess weight can be a sign of an endocrine abnormality or be simply due to excessive calorie intake.

Testing for endocrine imbalances

If you develop any one of these signs or symptoms, you should receive a complete endocrine and gynecologic evaluation. This evaluation requires specific blood tests and examinations that are usually done by your gynecologist or by an endocrinologist.

If you're an adult male who has acne, an endocrine evaluation is rarely performed. You may be asked about medications and hormonal supplements as well as general questions about your health and your sex life. In very rare occasions, your doctor may suspect an underlying disorder such as *adrenal hyperplasia* (see the section later in this chapter), and may order an endocrine evaluation. Make sure that you tell your doctor if you take any anabolic steroids because they can produce persistent acne in men.

If your dermatologist, gynecologist, or primary healthcare provider suspects androgen excess, he would probably order the following screening blood tests:

✔ **Free testosterone levels:** Elevations of free testosterone will often determine whether further testing is necessary. *Free testosterone* is the testosterone that's not bound to your sex hormone binding globulin (SHBG). When it's elevated, it can stimulate your acne-producing hair follicles and sebaceous glands. It is also "free" to cause other masculinizing signs and symptoms. For more on free testosterone and SHBG, see Chapter 11.

✔ **Dehydroepiandrosterone sulfate (DHEAS):** This chemical is used as a marker to see whether the adrenal glands are the source of excess androgen output.

These tests may determine if you have androgen excess and may provide clues to the origin of your excessive androgen production. If an abnormality is indicated by any of these blood tests as well as other sophisticated tests that may be out of the normal range, your doctor may recommend an evaluation by an *endocrinologist*. This doctor is a specialist in the study of the glands and hormones of the body and their related disorders (known as *endocrinology*). Alternatively, you may be referred to a gynecologist knowledgeable in endocrinology.

Considering the most common cause of androgen excess: PCOS

In females, *polycystic ovary syndrome* (PCOS) is the most common cause of androgen excess. The name comes from small cysts found in women's ovaries.

This disorder is characterized by menstrual irregularities, hirsutism, acne, ovarian cysts, varying degrees of insulin resistance, and often, obesity. Women with PCOS have a much higher risk of miscarriage. Many women are unaware that they have this disorder. PCOS has also been called *ovarian androgen excess* because the ovaries produce androgens in increased amounts. Because acne is influenced by androgens, it's not surprising that acne is a major symptom of PCOS.

Making the diagnosis

After reviewing your medical history and your family history, your physician will determine which tests are necessary. He may ask if you have been unable to become pregnant, or if there is type 2 diabetes in your family, which might make him more suspicious that you are more likely to have PCOS. Elevated androgen levels, DHEAS, or free testosterone, as I discuss earlier, help make the diagnosis of PCOS. The diagnosis is also aided by a physical exam and pelvic ultrasound (a noninvasive way to tell if you have ovarian cysts).

Most physicians will consider diagnosis of PCOS only after making sure you don't have other conditions such as Cushing's disease (overactive adrenal gland) or congenital adrenal hyperplasia — both of which are described later in this chapter.

One of the major features of PCOS is *insulin resistance.* This occurs when your body cells don't respond to even high levels of your own insulin. This causes *glucose* (sugar) to build up in the blood and can result in type 2 diabetes. (Type 2 diabetes used to be known as *adult onset* diabetes.) It's believed that the higher levels of blood insulin produce an increase in ovarian androgen production, particularly testosterone, and a decrease in concentrations of SHBG, the protein in charge of "mopping up" free testosterone (see Chapter 11).

Treating PCOS

Although this condition isn't curable, there are several approaches to correct the hormonal imbalance and symptoms of PCOS.

PCOS can be treated with medications used for the treatment of type 2 diabetes such as insulin-lowering therapy. Anti-androgen

Recognizing and treating PCOS

Angela, a 17-year-old girl, came to my office and told me about the difficulty that previous doctors had in managing her acne. Her mother said that Angela had still not gotten her first period and it was quite obvious that she was markedly over-weight. (She weighed 180 pounds and was only 5 feet tall.)

Angela's acne was severe and she had excessive hair growth on her face. It was apparent to me that she might have the endocrine abnormality known as polycystic ovary syndrome (PCOS) or another similar endocrine problem. I referred her to an endocrinologist, who, after obtaining a series of blood tests, diagnosed Angela as having PCOS. Her blood tests revealed that she had elevated androgens and evidence of insulin resistance. The endocrinologist started Angela on a medication that improved her sensitivity to insulin and she was also given anti-androgen hormones pills to take.

She lost 20 pounds; her periods began after six months of treatment, and her acne improved. The therapy also reduced some of her hirsutism. With the proper treatment, Angela has been able to live a normal life and now has two healthy children.

medications such as birth control pills, spironolactone, and flutamide have been shown to reverse the endocrine abnormalities seen with PCOS; these medications also help in decreasing hair loss, diminishing facial and body hair growth, normalizing the menstrual cycle, producing weight loss, and, of course, reducing acne lesions. These hormones are reviewed in Chapter 11.

Touching On Other Endocrine Disorders

Acne is a symptom of several hormonal disorders. They include congenital adrenal hyperplasia, Cushing's disease, and Cushing's syndrome. In all of these disorders, the body produces excess corticosteroids. These corticosteroids can have androgen-like activity. A detailed discussion of the features and treatment of these entities is beyond the scope of this book; however, I briefly describe them in the next few sections.

Congenital adrenal hyperplasia

Congenital adrenal hyperplasia (CAH) is caused by a missing *enzyme* (a protein that causes a chemical change in other substances without being changed itself) that your body needs to function properly. The missing enzyme results in an overproduction of male hormones (androgens).

The most common type of CAH results from low production of an enzyme of the adrenal gland called 21-hydroxylase. Mild forms of the disease (called nonclassical CAH) result in symptoms such as severe acne, excess facial and/or body hair (hirsutism), early development of pubic hair, receding scalp hairline, menstrual disturbances in females, and infertility in both males and females.

Cushing's disease and Cushing's syndrome

Acne, or more accurately, "acnelike" lesions, can be seen in Cushing's disease and Cushing's syndrome.

Cushing's disease is the name given to a condition caused by a pituitary tumor that secretes excessive amounts of *adrenocorticotropic hormone* (known as ACTH). This hormone stimulates the adrenal glands to produce excessive amounts of the hormone cortisol. Other tumors or conditions also may lead to excess secretion of cortisol such as tumors of the adrenal glands. This closely related disease is called *Cushing's syndrome*. Most often, Cushing's syndrome is caused by taking steroid hormones for long periods of time, particularly in high doses.

The symptoms include upper body obesity, a rounded ("moon") face, increased fat around the neck, and thinning arms and legs. Other symptoms include fatigue, weak muscles, high blood pressure, and high blood sugar.

Women usually have excess hair growth on their faces, necks, chests, abdomens, and thighs. Their menstrual periods may become irregular or stop. Men have decreased fertility with diminished or absent desire for sex.

The "acne" appears to be more akin to a folliculitis and consists of papules and pustules. Lesions usually arise on the chest and back and, in time, disappear when the oral cortisone is stopped, or when the levels of cortisone become normal after Cushing's disease and Cushing's syndrome are properly treated.

Blood and urine cortisol tests, together with the determination of adrenocorticotropic hormone (ACTH), are the three most important tests in the investigation of these conditions caused by an overproduction of cortisol.

Part V
The Part of Tens

The 5th Wave
By Rich Tennant

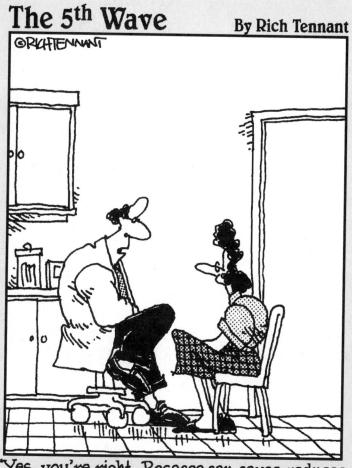

"Yes, you're right. Rosacea can cause redness in your face. The fact that this symptom only occurs when the pool boy is working in your backyard, however, raises some questions."

In this part . . .

Ah, the Part of Tens. It's like the icing on the cake. In this part, I provide you with ten great Web sites to learn more about acne and rosacea, I provide ten of my best tips for keeping your skin looking and feeling healthy, and I tell you about ten things that you should never do to your face. Enjoy.

Chapter 21

Ten Terrific Acne and Rosacea Web Sites

In This Chapter

▶ Searching the Internet

▶ Taking in the sites

*Y*ou can find a wide range of resources related to acne on the Internet. Many of them make fraudulent claims about their ability to "cure" your acne and are simply after your money. Instead of wandering aimlessly though the Web, I've done some clicking on my own for you and checked all of the sites that are mentioned in this chapter. They're chock-full of information and advice about acne and rosacea.

AcneNet

www.skincarephysicians.com/acnenet/index.html

This site is brought to you by the fine folks at the American Academy of Dermatology (www.aad.org), the largest of all dermatologic associations. It has a membership of more than 14,000 physicians worldwide. AcneNet is billed as "A comprehensive on-line acne information resource," and it lives up to its name. You can read more about tips, myths, and treatments, and you can locate a dermatologist in your area. Plus, if you back up the URL a bit to www.skincarephysicians.com, you can find all sorts of additional skin-care information and resources from the experts.

American Society for Dermatologic Surgeons

www.asds-net.org

The ASDS represents specialists in dermatologic surgery. This organization is comprised of experts in the diagnosis and surgical and cosmetic treatment of diseases of the skin, hair, and nails. This site can tell you about various procedures, technologies, and the latest techniques that are available to dermatologic surgeons. It also provides many helpful links for members and the general public to search for more information on dermatology, dermatologic surgery, and related topics on the Internet.

DermNet NZ

http://dermnetnz.org/acne

The New Zealand Dermatological Society sponsors this site used by both medical practitioners and consumers. Besides acne and rosacea, this site also has information about many other skin diseases and their treatment.

eMedicine.com

www.eMedicine.com

This site has a wealth of the most current information about diseases and disorders. It's available to physicians, other healthcare professionals, as well as the public. Nearly 10,000 physician authors (I'm one of them) and editors contribute to it.

The consumer health site, www.eMedicineHealth.com, contains articles written by physicians for the consumer. To access the acne information, simply scroll down to the "Topics" section and click on the "A" link, which brings you to the "Acne" link (along with links to all the other "A" conditions). There are also numerous links that tell you about the latest in health news.

MedLine Plus: Acne

www.nlm.nih.gov/medlineplus/acne.html

MedlinePlus is a service of the U.S. National Library of Medicine and the National Institutes for Health. On this site, you can find links to the latest acne news on acne treatments, various acne-related directories, and a skin-type calculator, among others. They also have an interactive acne tutorial. And if you've never checked out MedLine Plus (www.nlm.nih.gov/medlineplus), take a spin around the site — it has tons of information on whatever ails ya.

Omni: Acne Vulgaris

http://omni.ac.uk/browse/mesh/D000152.html

Omni is a U.K.-based Web catalog of Internet information on health and medicine. This site has a great deal of information and educational material about acne. Besides acne, it also has patient education handouts that cover other health-related problems.

RosaceaNet

www.skincarephysicians.com/rosaceanet

Also brought to you by the American Academy of Dermatology (see "AcneNet," earlier in the chapter), this site focuses on the signs, symptoms, and the latest treatments for rosacea.

Stop Spots

www.stopspots.org

This site for teens and young adults from U.K.-based Acne Support Group presents a number of top-ten lists, including their top ten acne tips, top ten beauty tips, and top ten problems folks with acne face. And you thought it was only the fabulous folks at *For Dummies* and a certain late-night talk show host that brought you great top ten lists!

Acne Support Group

www.m2w3.com/acne

Written in a user-friendly style, this U.K.-based site provides information and support for those who have acne or rosacea. It describes many of the facts and fictions about these skin conditions and it offers sensible advice about how to deal with them. It also has links to many other valuable sites.

Dermatology in the Cinema

www.skinema.com

This site is awesome! It's maintained by a dermatologist/film buff. It features images of skin conditions that have been depicted in the movies by using the Hollywood magic of makeup. It also has images of some of Hollywood's biggest stars that are shown with their real skin conditions — warts, acne, and all!

Chapter 22

Ten Tips for Healthy Skin

*T*hat's right. You don't see the word *acne* in the title of this chapter. And although the subject comes up here, it's not my primary focus. As a dermatologist, healthy skin is my thing. So, I wanted to provide you with some tips and tricks to keep your skin healthy throughout your life. Just think — you're going to get your acne under control one day, but you'll have the skin you're in for the rest of your life. So, treat it right. In this chapter, I show you how.

Steering Clear of Excessive Sun Exposure

The sun is an immense nuclear reactor. As well as producing heat and light, it also sends out other types of radiation that can sometimes damage your skin. The Earth's atmosphere filters out much of the more dangerous solar radiation, but some of it gets through — mainly in the ultraviolet (UV) band. The UV radiation in sunlight can cause painful sunburns and certain types of skin cancer, and can also age your skin.

If you have a personal or family history of skin cancer or you have very fair skin that never tans but always burns, do whatever possible to minimize sun exposure. If you have skin of color or are naturally very dark complexioned, you can probably ignore the following advice unless you develop allergic reactions from the sun, take medications that may make you extra sensitive to the sun, or have a medical condition that sunlight worsens.

The best way to prevent skin damage from the sun besides moving to the Antarctic — oops, never mind, I forgot about the hole in the ozone layer there — is to avoid excessive exposure to UV and the sun. You can accomplish this by following these tips:

- ✔ Shun the sun between 10 a.m. and 4 p.m, especially during late spring and summer when the sun is most intense.

- ✔ Wear protective headgear such as a hat with a wide brim to protect your face, head, and the back of your neck. You can also wear a baseball cap, long-sleeved shirts, and long pants.

- ✔ Be aware of reflected light from sand, water, or snow.

- ✔ Avoid tanning parlors.

- ✔ Slather on the sunscreen with an SPF of 15 or greater — at least 30 minutes before sun exposure, even on cloudy, hazy days.

- ✔ Reapply sunscreens liberally and frequently at least every two to three hours, and after swimming or sweating.

- ✔ Choose a broad spectrum sunscreen that blocks both UVB (the burning rays) and UVA (the more penetrating rays that promote wrinkling and aging).

If you're a person of color and have the dark spots of PIP, they're often further darkened by sun exposure. A broad-spectrum sunscreen will offer you the best protection. (I cover PIP in Chapter 12.)

Opting for Sunless Tanning

Sunless tanners, sometimes referred to as *self-tanners* or *tanning extenders,* are promoted as a way to get a tan without the sun. You can try:

- ✔ **Self-tanners:** These artificial tanning preparations contain dihydroxyacetone (DHA). DHA interacts with dead surface cells in the outermost (horny) layer of your epidermis and produces a color change. As the dead skin cells naturally slough off, the color gradually fades back to your normal skin color, typically within five to seven days after a single application. DHA-containing products are available as lotions, creams, sprays, and gels and aren't considered to be harmful. Airbrush tanning using DHA is now offered in salons.

- ✔ **Bronzers:** The term "bronzer" refers to a variety of products used to achieve a temporary tanned appearance. These products contain a transparent color additive that also stains the outermost layer of your skin. You can choose a bronzing gel or cream that enhances your own skin color. The chemicals in bronzers may react differently on various areas of your body, producing a tan of many shades. It can be washed off with soap and water at the end of each day. Bronzers are also considered to be harmless.

Although self-tanners and bronzers give the skin a golden brown color, these products don't offer protection from the damaging effects of UV radiation unless they also contain sunscreen ingredients.

Clinique, Estee Lauder, Clarins, and Bain de Soleil all offer sunless tanning products. Neutrogena has foams that are easy to apply to areas with body hair.

Other means of producing a tan without the sun, including tanning pills (which contain color additives) and tanning "accelerators" (which contain other chemicals), should be avoided. According to the FDA, there is a lack of scientific data showing that they work; in fact, at least one study has found them ineffective.

Dimming the Shine of Oily Skin

If you have oily skin — you're lucky! Oily skin has great advantages. Your skin will probably be less likely to wrinkle, age, and sag. On the other hand, it may feel greasy and develop shiny patches even a short time after you wash it. The highest concentration of sebaceous glands is in the T-zone, and the excess sebum from this area plus the sweat glands on the skin can make your skin look even greasier and shinier. (Take a look at Chapter 4 to see the T-zone.)

But you can temporarily squelch the shine with many products now available such as blotting papers, oil-absorbing powders, and foundations. Even the application of medicated prescription products such as retinoids and benzoyl peroxide are temporary cosmetic maneuvers that remove the surface oil. The deeper oils (sebum) are bound to keep flowing despite what you do to the surface.

You can try tackling T-zone oiliness with Clinac O.C. (Oil Control) Gel, which can be purchased without a prescription. It mops up excess sebum without drying the skin. In addition, if you're looking for a matte finish, you can try a "mattifier," a shine-stopping product that helps absorb oil on your face and, ideally, prevents oil from breaking through. The following are a few suggestions:

  ✔ Neutrogena Pore Refining Mattifier Shine Control Gel

  ✔ Lancome Pure Focus T-Zone Mattifier

  ✔ Loreal Hydra Mattify

Humidifying Dry Skin

If your skin is excessively dry, it may be due to a diminished production of sebum, reduced sweat activity, and environmental factors.

Xerosis, or dry skin, can affect anyone, but it tends to be more severe in certain folks, especially those with a hereditary predisposition. Modern lifestyles are also a contributing factor. In Western societies, we tend to over-bathe; use of harsh soaps and hot water also contribute. Xerosis is a common occurrence in winter climates, particularly in conditions of cold air, low relative humidity, and indoor heating.

Use moisturizers to help with dry skin. Moisturizers don't add water to the skin, but they help to retain or "lock in" water that was absorbed during your shower or bath. Therefore, apply a moisturizer while your skin is still damp. The choice of product is based on personal preference, ease of application, cost, and effectiveness.

 You can find numerous over-the-counter preparations in ointment bases, cream bases, and lotions. Eucerin, Nivea, Aquaphor, Oil of Olay, Moisturel, and Curel are just a few of the popular name brands. Am-Lactin (ammonium lactate 12 percent) lotion or cream is applied after bathing. It is very effective and is used for more severe cases of xerosis and may be purchased over the counter. If your skin is really scaly and dry, you can also get special, heavy-duty moisturizers that are available by prescription only.

Soothing Sensitive Skin

Acne medications, many of which are irritating in the first place, can wreak havoc with sensitive skin. Applying bland moisturizers such as Oil of Olay and Cetaphil Lotion *over* acne medications and using soap-free, gentle cleansers designed for sensitive skin is particularly important for people who have an underlying skin condition such as eczema (atopic dermatitis).

 Women who have sensitive skin or eczema should discard cosmetics that have been on the shelf for a long period. That's because they can become contaminated if some of their preservatives break down or oxidize over time.

Promoting a Youthful Glow

If you're looking for ways to promote that "youthful glow" of your skin, there are many new skin-care developments designed to do just that:

- ✔ **Renova:** Available only by prescription, this is an anti-aging cream that contains the active ingredient retinoic acid. Retinoic acid has been sold for years under the brand name Retin-A and used for the treatment of acne, which I cover in Chapter 9. The drug is approved by the FDA for the treatment of sun-damaged skin. Precautions for use of Renova are the same as those for tretinoin and the other retinoids.

- ✔ **Fruit acids:** Products that contain natural fruit acids (alpha hydroxy acids or AHAs) such as glycolic acid are now very popular. They claim to "rejuvenate" the skin by encouraging the shedding of old, sun-damaged surface skin cells, which promotes a fresher, healthier look with a more even color and texture. There are many products with varying concentrations of various fruit acids in differing bases. Those available from medical practitioners are stronger than those at pharmacies and beauty therapists. AHAs can be alternated with other topical anti-aging preparations including retinoid creams. Check out Chapter 14 where I talk more about AHAs.

Caring for the Bumps

Use the gentlest skincare products available if you have acne, rosacea, or razor bumps. Tender loving care is the byword. Treat your skin as gently as possible. Often, people suffer from their own overtreatment. Strong soaps, harsh exfoliants, loofahs, and rough washcloths are much too irritating.

Soap cleansers such as Basis soap, Eucerin Bar, Purpose Soap, and Neutrogena Cleansing Bar are all mild enough for daily washing.

Non-soap cleansers include Liquid Neutrogena Cleansing Formula, Aquinil Lotion, and Cetaphil Lotion.

Minimizing Stress

Easier said than done, I realize. Although stress doesn't cause acne, many believe that it can trigger flare-ups. That's because when the body encounters stress, it steps up production of cortisol, which causes the sebaceous glands to produce more oil.

The best course of action is to keep tabs on your own personal response, and to try to make time every day for the things that make you feel relaxed and happy. Exercise, meditate, get a good night's sleep, and eat a healthy diet. You've got nothing to lose.

Visiting a Dermatologist

If you may permit me to brag, we dermatologists have the important skills that come with focused, repetitive, visual scrutiny and education regarding your skin. The ability to make diagnoses and to identify benign versus malignant lesions is our specialty. And, of course, we're the experts when it comes to treating acne.

So if you can't manage your acne on your own or you're not getting very far with prescription medications given to you by your health-care provider, make an appointment to see one of us.

After you have a dermatologist, if you wake up one morning with a big zit and you have an important day coming up, call her office. Tell the person at the appointment desk about your problem. If it's during the week when your doctor has office hours, she'll be more likely than not to ask you to come in for an intralesional cortisone injection. It can flatten the bump within 24 to 48 hours. I describe this procedure in Chapter 10.

If that big day is today, do your best to hide the zit with makeup. Creative use of cosmetics can help conceal the redness of pimples, and green-tinted makeup can offer extra coverage.

Giving Yourself a Break

New products are constantly introduced to "correct" our "flaws," and draw us into an attempt to reach an impossible standard of beauty. Movies, advertisements, and TV present unrealistic images of youth and beauty in our image-obsessed culture. Infomercials, Internet ads, magazines, and yes, doctors, may promote — and sometimes exploit — the latest "miracle" cosmetic, diet, or plastic surgical techniques and promise you the "fountain of youth."

There is profound truth to the old proverbs — "beauty is only skin deep" and "it's what's inside that counts."

Relax and look at the glass as half full, rather than the idea that it is half empty. And remember — zits and pores get bigger the closer you look at them!

Chapter 23

Ten Things You Should Never Do to Your Skin

. . . .

In This Chapter

▶ Popping pimples is forbidden . . . most of the time

▶ Smoking is prohibited all of the time!

▶ Irritating your skin unnecessarily

▶ Resisting fly-by-night cures and the urge for instant gratification

. . . .

*Y*our skin is your protector that meets and greets your external world. As your body's largest organ, the skin serves as a waterproof covering that helps keep out foreign invaders and protects against temperature changes and sunlight. Your skin is tough and it can take a lot of punishment, but some things can make it look bad and weaken it. In this chapter, I review some actions that are harmful to your skin.

Picking, Popping, or Squeezing

Popping zits doesn't make things better; in fact, it often makes things worse. I realize that it's tempting to think that squeezing them will help them heal more quickly — especially the swollen, red goobers filled with stuff! But scrunching these guys only pushes the inflamed gunk deeper and wider into the skin and that's what most often results in scars. So, lay off the lumps! Having said all that, I realize that it's hard to resist a squeeze or two here and there, but only do so when dealing with blackheads and whiteheads.

If you're a do-it-yourselfer or plan to become a dermatologist or a cosmetologist, you can buy your own comedo extractor at a medical supply company. Better yet, see a dermatologist or go for a facial to have your blackheads and whiteheads extracted professionally.

Pre-tanning at a Salon

Pre-tanning at a tanning salon to get ready for the intense sun at the beach isn't the great idea that it's been cut out to be. In fact, whether you acquire a tan quickly or slowly, you still damage your skin. Just like the sun, artificial tanning equipment beds and sun lamps emit UV rays that can cause burns, premature aging, and skin cancers, especially if you're a higher risk, fair-skinned person who produces less melanin.

Smoking

You've heard about the risks of smoking (like lung cancer, heart disease, and emphysema). But have you ever noticed that the skin of elderly smokers tends to have a yellowish coloration? Next to sun exposure, smoking is the highest factor in wrinkling. In other words, smoking makes you look older!

The nicotine in cigarette smoke also causes small blood vessels and capillaries of the skin to contract. This diminishing circulation deprives the skin of much essential oxygen it needs to create and maintain healthy skin cells.

There's no controversy about this one — don't smoke!

Taking Too Much Vitamin A

You may have heard that vitamin A helps to cure acne. What you may not know is that if you take too much of it, vitamin A can accumulate in your liver to dangerous levels and cause serious health problems. Get your vitamin A from veggies. Good sources include leafy greens (like spinach and watercress) and orange veggies (like sweet potatoes, pumpkin, and carrots).

There are safer derivatives of vitamin A to treat your acne — topical retinoids and oral Accutane — that your healthcare provider can prescribe.

Traveling the Perilous Peel and Dermabrasion Route

If your complexion is dark, you may run the risk of having streaking, uneven pigmentation after chemical peel or dermabrasion procedures. Moreover, if you scar easily or tend to form keloids, you should probably consider these procedures as being potentially too risky.

Get a second or third opinion from practitioners experienced in these procedures on patients with your type of skin before embarking on something you might regret.

Treating Rosacea with Over-the-Counter Medications

Don't try to go it alone when you have rosacea. You should discuss your rosacea skin-care with a dermatologist. That's because folks who have rosacea tend to have red, inflamed, sensitive skin.

Consult with a dermatologist before experimenting with untried products. And definitely check out Chapter 18 for more tips on treating rosacea.

Applying Topical Steroids to Your Face

Okay, if you have a mild rash or itch, you can go to your local store and buy the over-the-counter, low-strength cortisone cream or ointment to treat the symptoms for a few days or so. However, don't make it a regular habit and use the stuff every day! It can cause acne and potentially thin your skin if you use it continuously.

You *definitely should not* use a potent prescription-strength topical steroid on your face without being instructed to by your doctor or dermatologist. Steroid-induced rosacea and skin thinning are much more likely to occur with the high potency spreads. Go to Chapter 18 to find out more about topical steroid-induced rosacea.

Shaving with Four-In-One Razor Blades

If you have acne, shaving bumps, or sensitive skin, those razors that guarantee the closest shaves aren't for you. Ignore the ongoing battle between razor companies to see who can stick the most blades on a single disposable razor head. Besides costing an arm and a leg, two, three, or four incredibly sharp blades will wind up shaving you two, three, or four more times closer than is necessary and really irritate your skin!

Easy does it. Let your hairs grow a little and when you do shave use a single blade safety razor such as the Aveeno PFB Bump Fighter Razor. I discuss razor bumps in Chapter 19.

Using Mystery Products

If it sounds too good to be true, it probably isn't true.

You may hear about alternative medications from friends, relatives, or the news media. Ads may suggest that alternative treatments can produce positive results in patients who have acne or rosacea.

Exercise caution — some of these drugs may have fraudulent claims, and others may even hurt you. Herbs can be as toxic and dangerous as prescription drugs. Look out for and avoid:

- ✔ "Secret" formulas (real scientists share what they know)

- ✔ Amazing breakthroughs or miracle cures (real breakthroughs don't happen every day, and when they do, real scientists don't call them "amazing' or "miracles")

- ✔ Guaranteed cures

The problem with herbal medications is that it's hard to know exactly what's in them because there is no regulation regarding their contents. For example, there have been reports of actual harm caused by St. John's wort, which has been found to make some people more sensitive to the sun.

Let your healthcare provider or dermatologist know about any of these products you may be taking or are considering taking.

There have been reports of severe toxic reactions, so you should be very cautious before trying anything that is untested.

Looking in the Mirror too Much

If you're undergoing treatment for your acne, you should know that it won't improve overnight and by examining it continuously, you just magnify any flaws — real or imagined.

When you apply makeup, use a "soft focus" with your eyes and don't take magnified close-up looks at your zits or comedones. You'll be amazed at how quickly your skin will improve if you ignore it for a few days at a time while your medications have a chance to work!

Part VI
Appendixes

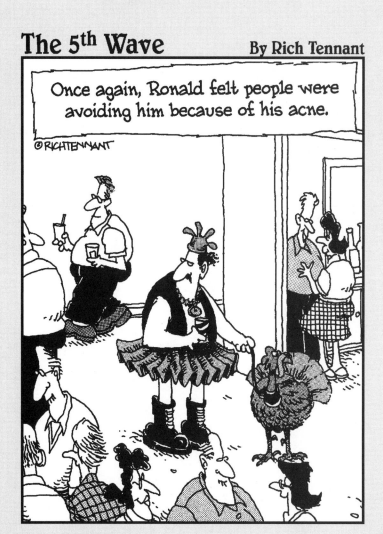

Once again, Ronald felt people were avoiding him because of his acne.

In this part . . .

1 provide you with some easily accessible and useful information that includes a glossary of terms you may run into at the dermatologist's office or the on the drug-store shelves and an international list of brand name acne medications.

Appendix A

Glossary

Accutane: Powerful drug derived from vitamin A that's used in the treatment of severe acne. The generic name is *isotretinoin.* If taken during pregnancy, it's highly likely to cause severe birth defects.

Acne: Skin condition characterized by plugging and inflammation that involves the *hair follicles* and *sebaceous glands.* It can take many forms including *blackheads, whiteheads, papules, pustules,* and *nodules.*

Acnegenic: Topical or oral products that produce or worsen acne lesions.

Acne vulgaris: Medical term for common acne.

Active ingredient: The chemical in a medication that does the work for which the product is designed.

Adult-onset acne: Overwhelmingly a condition of females, this type of acne turns up after the age of 18. It can crop up in a woman's 20s, 30s, or even later in life. It's sometimes referred to as *female adult acne* or *post-adolescent acne.*

Alpha hydroxy acids (AHAs): Fruit acids found in plants; constituents of many over-the-counter acne and cosmetic products, such as moisturizers and sunscreens. Also used in chemical peels.

Androgens: General term for *hormones* that have masculinizing features. Both males and females produce them. They cause the *sebaceous gland* to enlarge and produce more *sebum,* an important factor in the development of *acne.*

Antibiotic: Large category of drugs that has the ability to kill or inhibit the growth of bacteria.

Astringent: Solution that removes oil from the skin. Often used after a facial wash to remove any remaining traces of a cleanser.

Atrophy: A wasting away; a decrease in size of a tissue or body part.

Azelaic acid: Natural chemical produced by yeast. Used as a topical agent to treat *acne* and *rosacea*. It can also be used to lighten the skin.

Basal layer: The lowermost layer of the *epidermis*. This layer provides replacement cells that travel upward and replenish the skin with new cells.

Benzoyl peroxide: Topical antibacterial agent used to treat *acne*. Found in more over-the-counter and prescription products than any other topical agent.

Beta hydroxy acids (BHAs): A class of acids, including salicylic acid, that are used as exfoliants. They're found in many over-the-counter acne and cosmetic products, such as moisturizers and sunscreens. They're also used in *chemical peels*.

Blackhead: An *open comedo*. The dark acne *lesion* that consists of a plug of *keratin* and *sebum*. The dark color is due to a buildup of *melanin*.

Blue light therapy: Visible light treatment that works by killing the acne-producing bacteria, *P. acnes,* for a short period of time.

Chemical peel: Application of chemicals to the face in order to *exfoliate* the outer layer of skin cells.

Clindamycin: Topical *antibiotic* often used in the treatment of *acne.*

Closed comedo: *See whitehead.*

Collagen: Resilient protein that provides rigidity and strength to the *dermis.* Plays a major role in repairing damage to the skin and the development of all scars, including acne scars.

Comedo: Plug of *keratin* and *sebum* within a *hair follicle.* It can appear as a *blackhead* or a *whitehead.* The plural form is comedones.

Comedo extraction: A procedure performed with a round loop that's used to apply pressure to dislodge the contents of *blackheads* and *whiteheads.*

Comedogenic: Products that induce the formation of *comedones* (*blackheads* and *whiteheads*).

Comedogenesis: Medical term for the process that forms *whiteheads* and *blackheads.*

Comedolytic: Signifies that the product breaks up and inhibits *comedo* formation.

Comedonal acne: *See non-inflammatory acne.*

Contact dermatitis: Allergic reaction or irritant response to things that have touched your skin. Poison ivy and poison oak are classic examples.

Corticosteroid: Natural *hormones* produced in the adrenal glands. When used therapeutically, they are powerful anti-inflammatory drugs used to treat many types of *inflammation.*

Cyst: A fluid-filled mass that is usually benign. When someone has acne, the term *cyst* is often used interchangeably to mean *nodule* because of the resemblance of a nodular acne *lesion* to a cyst.

Depilatories: Creams, lotions, or powders that contain chemicals that split the chemical bonds in hair, breaking them off slightly below the surface of the skin.

Dermabrasion: Method to remove the skin's top layers and reduce acne scars using a rapidly rotating wheel or brush attached to a motorized handle to perform high-speed sanding. Newer technologies, such as lasers, have largely supplanted this procedure.

Dermatitis: Irritation or *inflammation* of the skin. A general term that refers to an itchy red rash. It is sometimes called *eczema.*

Dermis: Layer of the skin just beneath the *epidermis.* Contains blood and lymphatic vessels, *hair follicles,* nerves, and glands. Also called the *cutis.*

Doxycycline: An oral *tetracycline* antibiotic used to treat *acne* and *rosacea.*

Eczema: *See dermatitis.*

Elastin fibers: Found in the *dermis,* these protein structures are able to coil and recoil like a spring. They give the skin its elasticity.

Electrolysis: A permanent way to remove hair. It destroys hairs with electrical or thermal energy.

Emollient: Topical applications that are used to correct dryness and scaling of the skin.

Endocrine system: System of ductless glands that regulates bodily functions via *hormones* secreted into the bloodstream. Includes the hypothalamus, pituitary gland, thyroid, adrenal glands, and gonads (ovaries and testes).

Endocrinopathy: A disease of endocrine glands. A medical term for a hormonal disorder.

Enzymes: Proteins that cause a chemical change in other substances without being changed themselves.

Epidermis: Outer layer of the skin that lies upon the dermis.

Erector pilorum: *See hair erector muscle.*

Erythromycin: Oral and topical *antibiotic* that's often used in the treatment of *acne.*

Estrogen: Female *hormone* produced in the ovaries and adrenal glands.

Exfoliation: Removal of the outer layers of skin. It can be achieved with scrubs, glycolic and salicylic acids *(chemical peels),* as well as by *microdermabrasion.*

Fibroblasts: Cells that produce *collagen.*

Folliculitis: *Inflammation* of the *hair follicles.* It can be due to infections or eczema.

Hair canal: Part of the *hair follicle* through which *sebum* travels onto the hairs before it is carried out to the exterior of your skin.

Hair erector muscle (erector pilorum): Muscle connected to each *hair follicle* and the skin. When it contracts, it results in an erect hair and a goosebump on the skin.

Hair follicle: Tube-shaped covering that surrounds the part of the hair that is under the skin. Blockage of the follicle is produced by a follicular plug and is an important step in the formation of *acne.*

Heredity: Genetic transmission of a particular quality or trait from parent to offspring.

Hirsutism: Excessive growth of thick dark hair in locations where hair growth in women usually is minimal or absent. Usually occurs in *androgen*-stimulated locations, such as the face, chest, and around the nipples. May be a sign of *polycystic ovary syndrome* in women.

Hormones: The body's chemical messengers produced by the endocrine glands. They travel through the bloodstream and have specific effects on cells and organs in other parts of the body.

Hydroquinone: Chemical that's used to lighten (bleach) the skin.

Hyperpigmentation: Abnormal darkening of the skin that can follow *inflammation;* caused by higher amounts of *melanin* in a particular spot. It can also result from *hormones* and sun exposure.

Hypertrophic scar: Scars that bulge outward like hard lumps. The word *hypertrophy* means "enlargement" or "overgrowth."

Inflammation: A reaction of the skin to disease or injury.

Inflammatory acne: In this type of *acne, papules* or *pustules,* red or purple *macules,* and *nodules,* often termed "cysts," are predominant. There are few, if any, *comedones.*

Intense pulsed light treatment (IPL): Devices similar to lasers but use a wider range of wavelengths as opposed to only a single beam of light. They employ a broad band of visible and near infrared wavelengths of light that block out other wavelengths. It is hoped that they may able to affect the growth and activity of the *sebaceous gland* and help to treat *acne.*

iPLEDGE: An *isotretinoin* federal registry program geared toward reducing the number of birth defects, miscarriages, and abortions associated with isotretinoin. The registry keeps tabs on all isotretinoin prescriptions in the United States.

Isotretinoin: Chemical (generic) name for *Accutane.*

Keloid: Large scar whose size goes far beyond what would be expected from what seems to be a minor injury.

Keratin: Tough, fibrous protein that is inside the cells of the *epidermis.* It's also a constituent of hair and nails.

Keratinization: A process through which *keratinocytes* produce the protein *keratin.*

Keratinocytes: Make up the majority of the cells in the *epidermis.*

Keratosis pilaris: A condition of small, rough patches that tends to be mistaken for acne. It usually appears on the arms and sometimes on the cheeks.

Laser: Lasers produce single (concentrated) bands of light that can penetrate into the *dermis* without injuring the *epidermis.* They're used to treat *acne* and its scars. When used to treat acne, the beams are adjusted to penetrate below the epidermis and travel into the dermis where they can zero in on *hair follicles, sebaceous glands,* and the *P. acnes* bacteria.

Lesion: A mark in the skin. In dermatology, refers to a sore, growth, blister, or any other type of tissue damage caused by injury or disease.

Lipocytes: Fat cells.

Macule: Flat red, purple, or brown *lesion* that forms where a *papule* or *pustule* used to be. Remains visible for a while after an *acne lesion* has healed or is in the process of healing.

Melanin: Substance that gives the skin and hair its color and protects us against UV radiation.

Melanocyte: Cell in the *epidermis* that produces *melanin.*

Menopause: End of menstruation. The stage in life when women no longer have periods.

Menstruation: The periodic flow of blood from the uterus. Irregular *menses* can indicate a hormonal imbalance that can worsen *acne.*

Metronidazole: An antibiotic and antiparasitic drug that's used topically to treat *rosacea.*

Microcomedo: First stage of *comedo* formation; a comedo so small that it can be seen only with a microscope.

Microdermabrasion: Technique that uses aluminum oxide crystals passing through a vacuum tube to *exfoliate* surface skin.

Minocycline: An oral *tetracycline* antibiotic used to treat *acne* and *rosacea.*

Nodule: A large and lumpy, pus-filled, frequently reddish bump that is lodged more deeply in the skin. They are *inflammatory lesions* that are sometimes referred to as *cysts.*

Noncomedogenic: Skin-care products that have been tested and proven not to clog pores and produce *comedones.*

Noncomedonal acne: *See inflammatory acne.*

Non-inflammatory acne: This category of *acne* is identified when a person's *lesions* are primarily *whiteheads* and *blackheads.* It is also called *comedonal acne.*

Ocular rosacea: Rosacea that involves the eyes.

Open comedo: *See blackhead.*

Oral contraceptives: Drugs used to help prevent an unwanted pregnancy. If you're female, your doctor may also prescribe them to fight *acne* by virtue of their anti-androgenic effects.

Oral therapy: Something that's taken by mouth such as a pill, capsule, or liquid.

Papule: Pimples (zits) that appear as small, firm, reddish bumps on the skin. They are *inflammatory lesions.*

Perimenopause: The transitional period from normal menstrual periods to no periods at all.

Perioral dermatitis: Also known as *periorificial dermatitis*, this condition is a *rosacea*-like skin eruption seen almost exclusively in young women.

Pilosebaceous unit: Grouping of the *hair follicle* and its attached *sebaceous gland.*

Polycystic ovary syndrome: PCOS is characterized by menstrual irregularities, *hirsutism, acne,* ovarian cysts, varying degrees of insulin resistance, and often, obesity.

Pomade acne: Type of acne is seen in African-Americans and other individuals who have tight curly hair and frequently use pomade (oils and greasy ointments) to style or improve their hair's manageability.

Pores: The openings of *hair follicles* onto the skin. Through them, sweat and *sebum* flow onto the skin.

Postinflammatory hyperpigmentation: These dark spots are also called postinflammatory pigmentation, or PIP, for short. The original insult (and injury) that caused PIP can be a cut, a burn, a rash, or the after-effect from a healing *acne lesion.* The dark spots are limited to the sites of previous *inflammation.*

Prednisone: Synthetic *corticosteroid* that's used to treat inflammatory conditions.

Progesterone: Female *hormone* produced by the ovaries after ovulation to prepare the uterus for fertilization.

Progestin: Synthetic *progesterone.*

Propionibacterium acnes *(P. acnes):* These bacteria are an integral part of producing the *inflammatory lesions* of *acne.* They live in the pilosebaceous glands of the skin.

Pseudofolliculitis barbae (razor bumps): Acnelike *lesions* that occur mainly on the beard area in men of African heritage. This condition is due to curly, ingrown hairs.

Pulse dye laser (PDL): This laser is "tuned" to a specific wavelength of light. It produces a bright light that is absorbed by the superficial blood vessels of the skin. The abnormal blood vessels are destroyed without damaging the surrounding skin. This laser has been used to successfully treat acne scars and *rosacea telangiectasias.*

Punch excision: Surgical technique that's sometimes used to cut out and reduce certain types of acne scars.

Pustule: A papule that contains pus. It's also known as a *pus pimple.* An *inflammatory lesion.*

Resorcinol: A weakly acidic organic chemical obtained from various resins; found in some topical agents used to treat *acne.*

Retinoids: Chemicals related to vitamin A. A mainstay in the treatment of both *comedonal* and *inflammatory acne.* The major retinoids are Retin-A, tretinoin, Tazorac, and Differin.

Retention hyperkeratosis: Excessive buildup of skin cells that, combined with *sebum* and trapped bacteria, creates a plug in *hair follicles* that results in *acne lesions.*

Rhinophyma: Enlarged nose that results from enlarged *sebaceous glands* and overgrowth of *collagen,* and is a feature of *rosacea* that's seen primarily in men.

Rosacea: Acnelike condition characterized by redness, *papules,* and sometimes *pustules* in the center one third of the face in certain fair-complexioned adults. It's often mistaken for *acne.*

Salicylic acid: Ingredient found in many over-the-counter *acne* products. Helps to *exfoliate* the outer layers of the skin.

Sebaceous duct: Tiny tube that steers the *sebum* (and the dead skin cells it carries) from the *sebaceous* gland into the *hair canal.*

Sebaceous glands: Located in the *dermis* next to *hair follicles,* these are small, sack-shaped glands that release *sebum* onto the hair and moisturize the skin.

Sebum: Oily substance produced by *sebaceous glands* that coats the hair and skin. Composed of a rich blend of different *lipids* (fatty chemicals). Helps to keep the skin lubricated and protected. Clogs *pores,* helping to cause outbreaks of *acne.*

Sex hormone binding globulin: A protein in the blood that "mops up" free *testosterone* and prevents it from stimulating acne-producing oil glands to produce excess oil.

Spironolactone: An anti-androgen medication sometimes used in combination with *oral contraceptives* to treat *acne* in women.

Stratum corneum: Also known as the horny layer, it is the outermost layer of the *epidermis.* It is comprised of dead skin cells that protect deeper cells from damage, infection, and from drying out.

Stratum spinosum: This is the middle ("spiny") layer of the *epidermis.* These cells are always actively dividing.

Subcutaneous layer: Fatty layer of tissue located under the *dermis.*

Sulfacetamide: Anti-infective used topically to treat *acne* and *rosacea.* Often combined with sulfur.

Telangiectasias: Small, dilated blood vessels usually seen on the face. Also called broken blood vessels, or "spider veins."

Teratogenic: Drug that, if taken during pregnancy, is highly likely to cause severe birth defects.

Testosterone: An *androgen* and the main male *hormone.* Produced by the testes in men and by the ovaries in women.

Tetracycline: Oral antibiotic typically used to treat *acne* and *rosacea.*

Topical therapy: Something that's applied onto the skin, such as a cream, gel, or ointment.

Vehicle: Part of a product that holds the *active ingredient.* It's the base (ointment, gel, or cream) to which a medication is added.

Whitehead: Small, pearly white *acne lesion* that consists of a plug of *keratin* and *sebum.* Occurs when the *comedo* stays below the surface of the skin. Also called a *closed comedo.*

Appendix B

International Brand Names for Some of the Medications Listed in This Book

● ●

Table B-1			Topical Medications			
Generic Name	*United States*	*France*	*Germany*	*U.K.*	*Canada*	*Australia*
Adapalene	Differin	Differine	Differin	Differin	Differin	Differin
Azelaic acid	Azelex, Finacea	Skinoren, Finevin	Skinoren, Finevin	Skinoren, Finevin	Finacea	Skinoren
Benzoyl peroxide	Oxy-5, Oxy-10	PanOxyl, Eclaran	Benzaknen, PanOxyl, Benzoyt	PanOxyl, Acnecide	Benzac, PanOxyl	Benzac, Brevoxyl
Clindamycin	Cleocin-T	Dalacine T	Basocin	Dalacin T	Dalacin T	Clindatech
Erythromycin	Emgel, Staticin, Akne-Mycin	Eryacne, Eryfluid, Stimycine	Aknemycin, Stiemycine, Erythrocin	Stiemycin, Erymax, Eryacne	Erysol, Erythrocin, Staticin	Eryacne, Ilosone, Erythrocin
Metronidazole	Noritate, Metro-Gel, Metro-Cream	Rosiced, Rozagel	MetroGel	Rozex	MetroGel, Noritate	Rozex
Tazarotene	Tazorac	Zorac	Zorac	Zorac	Tazorac	Zorac
Tretinoin	Retin-A, Avita	Retin-A, Aberel, Effederm	Epi-Aberel, Eudyna	Retin-A	Retin-A, Vitinoin, Retisol-A	Retin-A, Stieva-A

Table B-2

Oral Medications

Generic Name	United States	France	Germany	U.K.	Canada	Australia
Doxycycline Hyclate	Vibramycin, Monodox, Vibra-Tabs, Adoxa	Vibramycine, Doxycycline	Vibramycin, Doxycycline	Vibramycin	Vibramycin, Vibra-Tabs, Doryx, Doxycin	Vibramycin, Vibra-Tabs, Doryx
Minocycline	Minocin, Dynacin	Mestacine, Mynocine	Skid, Lederderm	Minocin, Aknemin	Minocin	Minomycin
Erythromycin	E-Mycin, EES, Erythrocin	Erythrocyne	Erythrocin, Monomycin	Erythrocin, Erymax, Ilosone	E-Mycin, EES, Erythrocin	EES, Erythrocin, Ilosone
Isotretinoin	Accutane, Sotret, Amnesteem, Claravis	Roaccutane	Roaccutan	Roaccutane	Accutane	Accure, Roaccutane

Index

pore cleansing strips, 83
pores, 30–31, 275
post-adolescent acne, 269. *See also*
    adult-onset acne
postules, 50, 67
prednisone, 276
pregnancy
    acne during, 54–55
    birth defects and, 58, 105
    medication safety and, 55–57, 124
    tests, 157–158
pre-tanning, 262
primary healthcare provider (PCP)
    establishing treatment goals, 87–88
    providing referral to see a specialist,
        90–91
    types of, 88–89
    working with, 89
Princess Diana (British royalty), 218
professional associations, 92
professionals. *See* healthcare
    professionals; primary healthcare
    provider (PCP)
progesterone
    androgenic effects of, 52
    described, 29, 45, 276
    pregnancy and, 54
    puberty and, 45
    synthetic (progestin), 131, 276
Propionibacterium acnes. *See P. acnes*
pseudofolliculitis barbae (PFB)
    acne versus, 16, 51
    benzoyl peroxide treatments for,
        235–237
    causes of, 230–231
    described, 229, 276
    hair removal and, 237–240
    self treatment for, 233–235
    shaving and, 231–233
    slowing down hair growth and, 240
PSU (pilosebaceous unit), 27, 275
psychological scars
    adult-onset acne and, 52–53
    coping with, 204–205
    depression, 164–166, 205–206, 208
    emotional disorders, 209
    helping teenagers with, 206–208
    overview, 15, 203
    therapy for, 210
psychotherapy, 210
puberty, 29, 44, 45, 46
pulse therapy, 125
pulsed dye laser (PDL), 171, 276
pulsed light and heat energy (LHE), 171

punch excision, 276
pustules, 33, 213, 230, 276

• *Q* •

quackwatch (Web site), 15

• *R* •

radio wave therapy, 168, 202
razor bumps. *See* pseudofolliculitis
    barbae (PFB)
Rembrandt (Dutch painter), 218
Renova (anti-aging cream), 259
resorcinol, 82, 276
retention hyperkeratosis, 276
retinoids. *See also* isotretinoin
    applying, 105–106
    benefits of, 103–104
    brand name and generic, 104–105
    building up tolerance, 106
    chemical peels and, 173
    for comedonal acne, 36, 103
    described, 104, 276
    enhancing treatments and, 107
    for long-term maintenance, 103
    for postinflammatory
        hyperpigmentation (PIP), 145
    pregnancy and, 57, 105
    rosacea and, 222
    side effects, 106–107
    when to expect improvement, 105
retinols, 81
rhinophyma, 214, 227, 276
rosacea
    acne versus, 16, 215
    alcoholic beverages and, 220
    camouflaging the redness, 225–227
    causes/triggers of, 216–217, 219–221
    celebrities with, 218
    cosmetics and, 217–219, 225–226
    described, 51, 211, 276
    doxycycline for, 124
    look-alikes, 227–228
    metronidazole for, 223, 224, 274
    ocular rosacea, 214
    rhinophyma and, 214, 227
    self treatment and, 263
    skin conditions versus, 215–216
    steroid-induced, 67, 263
    symptoms of, 212–216
    treatments for, 221–225
    washing your face and, 217
    Web sites, 253, 254
RosaceaNet (Web site), 253

BUSINESS, CAREERS & PERSONAL FINANCE

0-7645-5307-0

0-7645-5331-3 *†

Also available:

Accounting For Dummies †
0-7645-5314-3

Business Plans Kit For Dummies †
0-7645-5365-8

Cover Letters For Dummies
0-7645-5224-4

Frugal Living For Dummies
0-7645-5403-4

Leadership For Dummies
0-7645-5176-0

Managing For Dummies
0-7645-1771-6

Marketing For Dummies
0-7645-5600-2

Personal Finance For Dummies *
0-7645-2590-5

Project Management For Dummies
0-7645-5283-X

Resumes For Dummies †
0-7645-5471-9

Selling For Dummies
0-7645-5363-1

Small Business Kit For Dummies *†
0-7645-5093-4

HOME & BUSINESS COMPUTER BASICS

0-7645-4074-2

0-7645-3758-X

Also available:

ACT! 6 For Dummies
0-7645-2645-6

iLife '04 All-in-One Desk Reference For Dummies
0-7645-7347-0

iPAQ For Dummies
0-7645-6769-1

Mac OS X Panther Timesaving Techniques For Dummies
0-7645-5812-9

Macs For Dummies
0-7645-5656-8

Microsoft Money 2004 For Dummies
0-7645-4195-1

Office 2003 All-in-One Desk Reference For Dummies
0-7645-3883-7

Outlook 2003 For Dummies
0-7645-3759-8

PCs For Dummies
0-7645-4074-2

TiVo For Dummies
0-7645-6923-6

Upgrading and Fixing PCs For Dummies
0-7645-1665-5

Windows XP Timesaving Techniques For Dummies
0-7645-3748-2

FOOD, HOME, GARDEN, HOBBIES, MUSIC & PETS

0-7645-5295-3

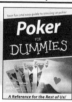

0-7645-5232-5

Also available:

Bass Guitar For Dummies
0-7645-2487-9

Diabetes Cookbook For Dummies
0-7645-5230-9

Gardening For Dummies *
0-7645-5130-2

Guitar For Dummies
0-7645-5106-X

Holiday Decorating For Dummies
0-7645-2570-0

Home Improvement All-in-One For Dummies
0-7645-5680-0

Knitting For Dummies
0-7645-5395-X

Piano For Dummies
0-7645-5105-1

Puppies For Dummies
0-7645-5255-4

Scrapbooking For Dummies
0-7645-7208-3

Senior Dogs For Dummies
0-7645-5818-8

Singing For Dummies
0-7645-2475-5

30-Minute Meals For Dummies
0-7645-2589-1

INTERNET & DIGITAL MEDIA

0-7645-1664-7

0-7645-6924-4

Also available:

2005 Online Shopping Directory For Dummies
0-7645-7495-7

CD & DVD Recording For Dummies
0-7645-5956-7

eBay For Dummies
0-7645-5654-1

Fighting Spam For Dummies
0-7645-5965-6

Genealogy Online For Dummies
0-7645-5964-8

Google For Dummies
0-7645-4420-9

Home Recording For Musicians For Dummies
0-7645-1634-5

The Internet For Dummies
0-7645-4173-0

iPod & iTunes For Dummies
0-7645-7772-7

Preventing Identity Theft For Dummies
0-7645-7336-5

Pro Tools All-in-One Desk Reference For Dummies
0-7645-5714-9

Roxio Easy Media Creator For Dummies
0-7645-7131-1

* Separate Canadian edition also available
† Separate U.K. edition also available

Available wherever books are sold. For more information or to order direct: U.S. customers visit www.dummies.com or call 1-877-762-2974.
U.K. customers visit www.wileyeurope.com or call 0800 243407. Canadian customers visit www.wiley.ca or call 1-800-567-4797.

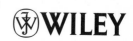

SPORTS, FITNESS, PARENTING, RELIGION & SPIRITUALITY

0-7645-5146-9

0-7645-5418-2

Also available:
- Adoption For Dummies
  0-7645-5488-3
- Basketball For Dummies
  0-7645-5248-1
- The Bible For Dummies
  0-7645-5296-1
- Buddhism For Dummies
  0-7645-5359-3
- Catholicism For Dummies
  0-7645-5391-7
- Hockey For Dummies
  0-7645-5228-7

- Judaism For Dummies
  0-7645-5299-6
- Martial Arts For Dummies
  0-7645-5358-5
- Pilates For Dummies
  0-7645-5397-6
- Religion For Dummies
  0-7645-5264-3
- Teaching Kids to Read
  For Dummies
  0-7645-4043-2
- Weight Training For Dummies
  0-7645-5168-X
- Yoga For Dummies
  0-7645-5117-5

TRAVEL

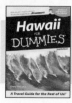

0-7645-5438-7

0-7645-5453-0

Also available:
- Alaska For Dummies
  0-7645-1761-9
- Arizona For Dummies
  0-7645-6938-4
- Cancún and the Yucatán
  For Dummies
  0-7645-2437-2
- Cruise Vacations For Dummies
  0-7645-6941-4
- Europe For Dummies
  0-7645-5456-5
- Ireland For Dummies
  0-7645-5455-7

- Las Vegas For Dummies
  0-7645-5448-4
- London For Dummies
  0-7645-4277-X
- New York City For Dummies
  0-7645-6945-7
- Paris For Dummies
  0-7645-5494-8
- RV Vacations For Dummies
  0-7645-5443-3
- Walt Disney World & Orlando
  For Dummies
  0-7645-6943-0

GRAPHICS, DESIGN & WEB DEVELOPMENT

0-7645-4345-8

0-7645-5589-8

Also available:
- Adobe Acrobat 6 PDF
  For Dummies
  0-7645-3760-1
- Building a Web Site For Dummies
  0-7645-7144-3
- Dreamweaver MX 2004
  For Dummies
  0-7645-4342-3
- FrontPage 2003 For Dummies
  0-7645-3882-9
- HTML 4 For Dummies
  0-7645-1995-6
- Illustrator CS For Dummies
  0-7645-4084-X

- Macromedia Flash MX 2004
  For Dummies
  0-7645-4358-X
- Photoshop 7 All-in-One Desk
  Reference For Dummies
  0-7645-1667-1
- Photoshop CS Timesaving
  Techniques For Dummies
  0-7645-6782-9
- PHP 5 For Dummies
  0-7645-4166-8
- PowerPoint 2003 For Dummies
  0-7645-3908-6
- QuarkXPress 6 For Dummies
  0-7645-2593-X

NETWORKING, SECURITY, PROGRAMMING & DATABASES

0-7645-6852-3

0-7645-5784-X

Also available:
- A+ Certification For Dummies
  0-7645-4187-0
- Access 2003 All-in-One Desk
  Reference For Dummies
  0-7645-3988-4
- Beginning Programming
  For Dummies
  0-7645-4997-9
- C For Dummies
  0-7645-7068-4
- Firewalls For Dummies
  0-7645-4048-3
- Home Networking For Dummies
  0-7645-42796

- Network Security For Dummies
  0-7645-1679-5
- Networking For Dummies
  0-7645-1677-9
- TCP/IP For Dummies
  0-7645-1760-0
- VBA For Dummies
  0-7645-3989-2
- Wireless All In-One Desk Reference
  For Dummies
  0-7645-7496-5
- Wireless Home Networking
  For Dummies
  0-7645-3910-8

HEALTH & SELF-HELP

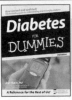

0-7645-6820-5 *†   0-7645-2566-2

Also available:

✔ Alzheimer's For Dummies
0-7645-3899-3

✔ Asthma For Dummies
0-7645-4233-8

✔ Controlling Cholesterol For Dummies
0-7645-5440-9

✔ Depression For Dummies
0-7645-3900-0

✔ Dieting For Dummies
0-7645-4149-8

✔ Fertility For Dummies
0-7645-2549-2

✔ Fibromyalgia For Dummies
0-7645-5441-7

✔ Improving Your Memory For Dummies
0-7645-5435-2

✔ Pregnancy For Dummies †
0-7645-4483-7

✔ Quitting Smoking For Dummies
0-7645-2629-4

✔ Relationships For Dummies
0-7645-5384-4

✔ Thyroid For Dummies
0-7645-5385-2

EDUCATION, HISTORY, REFERENCE & TEST PREPARATION

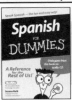

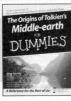

0-7645-5194-9   0-7645-4186-2

Also available:

✔ Algebra For Dummies
0-7645-5325-9

✔ British History For Dummies
0-7645-7021-8

✔ Calculus For Dummies
0-7645-2498-4

✔ English Grammar For Dummies
0-7645-5322-4

✔ Forensics For Dummies
0-7645-5580-4

✔ The GMAT For Dummies
0-7645-5251-1

✔ Inglés Para Dummies
0-7645-5427-1

✔ Italian For Dummies
0-7645-5196-5

✔ Latin For Dummies
0-7645-5431-X

✔ Lewis & Clark For Dummies
0-7645-2545-X

✔ Research Papers For Dummies
0-7645-5426-3

✔ The SAT I For Dummies
0-7645-7193-1

✔ Science Fair Projects For Dummies
0-7645-5460-3

✔ U.S. History For Dummies
0-7645-5249-X

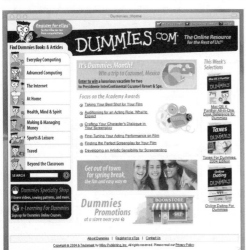

Get smart @ dummies.com®

- **Find a full list of Dummies titles**
- **Look into loads of FREE on-site articles**
- **Sign up for FREE eTips e-mailed to you weekly**
- **See what other products carry the Dummies name**
- **Shop directly from the Dummies bookstore**
- **Enter to win new prizes every month!**

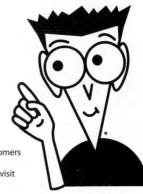

* Separate Canadian edition also available
† Separate U.K. edition also available

Available wherever books are sold. For more information or to order direct: U.S. customers visit www.dummies.com or call 1-877-762-2974.
U.K. customers visit www.wileyeurope.com or call 0800 243407. Canadian customers visit www.wiley.ca or call 1-800-567-4797.

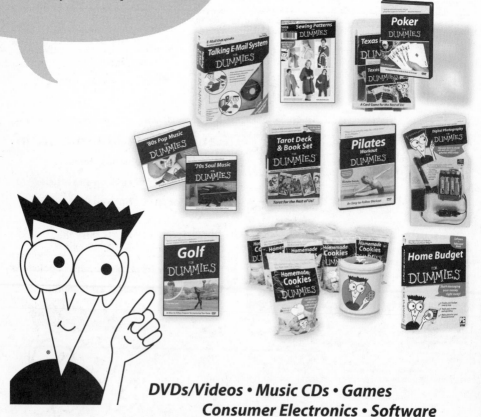
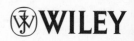